To: B_____ _____
With ___ _____ ___de
for your healing
presence, to so
many in need.
Every Nurse Matters!
E

The Ecology of Wellness for Nurses

Sharon Olson

2012

Other Books by Sharon Olson

Your Gift: An Educational, Spiritual, and Personal Resource for Hospice Volunteers
1987, Seasons Press, second edition 2000, third (25th Anniversary) edition 2012

Into the Light: For Women Experiencing the Transformative Nature of Grief
1993, Seasons Press

With Love from Old Mission: A Collection of Original Songs, Poetry, and Photography
1998, Seasons Press

The Ecology of Wellness for Nurses

A Personal and Professional Resource

Sharon Olson, Ph.D., GNP-BC

SEASONS PRESS
Traverse City, MI

© 2012 Seasons Press

Published by
Seasons Press
Traverse City, MI

Publisher's Cataloging-in-Publication Data
Olson, Sharon L.

The ecology of wellness for nurses : a personal and professional resource/ Sharon L. Olson. – Traverse City, MI : Seasons Press, 2012.

p. ; cm.

ISBN13: 978-0-9638984-6-3

1. Nursing—Philosophy. 2. Nursing models. 3. Nursing—Psychological aspect. I. Title.

RT84.5.O47 2012
610.7301—dc23   2012941458

FIRST EDITION

Project coordination by Jenkins Group, Inc.
www.BookPublishing.com

"Faith," © Patrick Overton used with permission, *Rebuilding the Front Porch of America*, 1997.

Front cover design by Lindsey Klintworth, Snap! Printing, Traverse City, MI
Interior design by Yvonne Fetig Roehler

Printed in the United States of America
16   15   14   13   12   •   5   4   3   2   1

In memory of Estyln Harms,
who helped me see.

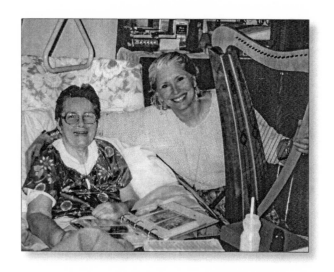

When we have done the best we can—
    When our hearts know the path—
When our spirits show the way—
    If only one person is touched—
That is enough—
    That is the blessing.
                        JOHN M. SCHNEIDER

CONTENTS

PREFACE

This is a small book with a collective big heart. I offer it to nurses as a way of "giving back" to a profession that has given me so much for almost half a century.

My experience with acute, chronic, and terminal illness has been rich and varied, and my brief military service as a young army nurse caring for severely wounded soldiers younger than myself profoundly reinforced my decision to become a nurse. As happened for me, I believe all nurses have, or will have, their own epiphanies regarding the direction their life's work will take.

Today, my path points me toward a new emphasis for nurses in the time that remains. One that commits me to helping you focus on your own wellness from a holistic ecological perspective. I believe now more than ever that our profession needs to re-connect and re-infuse its mission beyond the escalating skill sets required to treat illness. Now more than ever, we need to call ourselves back to what it means to be a healing presence—first and foremost to ourselves—in order that we can be truly present for our patients.

Regardless of what drew us to nursing, ultimately we committed our "whole selves" to steadfastly representing humanity on behalf of another human being. It is written in fine print at the bottom of our contract with life! How we embrace and uphold this responsibility is by continually monitoring the pulse of our own wellness—mind, body, and spirit. This is tantamount in discerning our caring from care. It holds us to the path of compassion for ourselves, our patients, and our loved ones.

Recently, I reviewed a very lengthy 2011 document entitled *The Future of Nursing, Leading Change, Advancing Health* from the Robert Wood Johnson Foundation Initiative on the Future of Nursing at the Institute of Medicine. It posited that as a profession we:

- Are poised to help bridge the gap between coverage and access as well as to coordinate increasingly complex care for a wide range of patients
- Are crucial in preventing medication errors, reducing rates of infection, facilitating and coordinating patient transitions into different care locations, and promoting health and wellness with reliable improvement of health outcomes tied to quality care measures and patient-centered care
- Provide compassionate care across the life span

This well-intentioned document reminds me of a quote by Rachel Naomi Remen, M.D., from her book *My Grandfather's Blessings*:

> In a highly technological world we may forget our own goodness and place value instead on our skills and our expertise. But it is not our expertise that will restore the world. The future may depend less on our expertise than on our faithfulness to life.

For the cover of this book, I deliberately chose a Pima Indian labyrinth design that my dear husband mowed into our meadow many years ago. Our labyrinth was open for people to walk at any time and in any season.

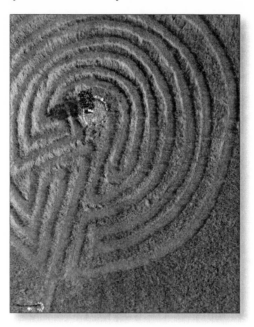

Originating over four thousand years ago, labyrinths were interwoven with sacred traditions across the world. Unlike a maze, a labyrinth offers only one path—always forward to the center—and is used as a reflective tool in both regrounding us to what we are about and reconnecting us to our own center of what is yet possible.

My hope is that this book will be a personal reflective resource for renewing your center of compassion. May the inspiring words contributed by your sisters and brothers in this profession keep your vision always forward on the path of caring.

ACKNOWLEDGMENTS

It is with deep gratitude that I thank the many nurses and nursing students who contributed inspiring pearls of wisdom to *The Ecology of Wellness for Nurses: A Personal and Professional Resource*. They profoundly validate the "why" in my decision to write this last book by conveying the width and depth of what remains essential for our profession.

Also, I am very grateful for Rebecca Chown, a pearl of wisdom in her own right, who has journeyed with me over many years with various writing projects. Her intuitive editorial expertise is more than remarkable. She also gently guides and encourages many individuals through their writing process to fully express their own truth.

With deep respect and gratitude, these chapters acknowledge and highlight a number of theorists who have been "terra firma" on my own personal and professional labyrinth walk. Their theoretical perspectives, perhaps written a number of years ago, became even more relevant as I developed my ecological model of wellness.

I particularly want to acknowledge Dr. John Schneider, a clinical psychologist who taught, wrote, and worked extensively in the area of grief and loss. Wordlessly, he helped me to truly "see" with new eyes the fullness of caring. I was blessed to share his compassionate life as both colleague and wife for many years. Daily, I saw him "walk his talk" about holding hope for individuals and validating both joys and sorrows while believing their "best self" would ultimately find what was yet possible. John's healing presence with individuals was palpably conveyed through silence, words, deeds, and even laughter.

Maya Angelou succinctly writes, "People will forget what you said—will forget what you did—but will never forget how you made them feel."

Let us endeavor to acknowledge, teach, and grow what is most essential to healing and wellness holistically. The future of nursing depends on it.

Sharon Olson
New Years Eve, 2011

Introduction:
Stepping Stones of Life
and Nursing Practice

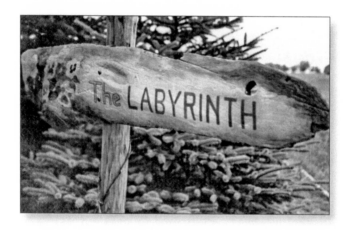

*The inner life of any great thing will be incomprehensible
to me until I develop and deepen an inner life of my own.*
Parker J. Palmer, in *The Book of Awakening*
by Mark Nepo

I realize it is a bold endeavor to offer yet another holistic
perspective of caring for nurses to consider, but it has always
been my nature to introduce new paths that lead toward what
I see as possible for this profession, paths that help me answer
the question, "What is the greater whole of the self in nursing?"

Now more than ever, nurses need philosophical and theoretical stepping stones that are both congruent with and a reflection of our personal values because nursing is more than just a job—it is a way of our being in this world for both men and women. I say this because the reality of today is that our professional dialogue now includes new terms such as "horizontal hostility," "lateral violence," "nurse-to-nurse bullying" or "sabotage," and "nurses eating their young." This overt and covert negativity is also perpetuated through witnesses who silently disagree with the offender but say nothing in defense of the recipient of the verbal abuse.

What has happened to bring us down this path? And I do mean down! From my perspective, it begins with spiritual discouragement. When our inner guide speaks its truth, we fail to act on that wisdom. Also, negative workplace experiences cause us to slowly loosen the firm grip of our nursing ideals and begin grasping resentment. We begin holding it tightly at work, at home, and even towards strangers over small injustices. We may become strangers even unto ourselves, leaving us asking, "Where is that kind and caring person I used to be?"

The good news is that with encouragement and self-validation, we can re-plant new seeds of compassion, gratitude, and healing presence for ourselves and our patients.

I recently watched a short YouTube video created by Kathleen Bartholomew, R.N., M.S.N. The author of *Ending Nurse-to-Nurse Hostility*, she is well known for eloquently calling nurses back to finding their voices and building positive work environment relationships that build on gratitude and clarity of purpose. In the video, which is available via her website at *www.kathleenbartholomew.com*, she shares a tender story about an experience she had while bathing a patient and then closes by offering gratitude to all nurses for "standing at the core of humanity."

When we remember that we do indeed stand at the core of humanity, our hearts open and our healing presence—for ourselves and for those we care for—is made manifest.

CIRCLES OF HEALING

As suggested in the Preface, I use a labyrinth metaphor to affirm both our personal and professional journeys. Each of us must find paths that continually renew and replenish our compassion and what it means to be a healing presence for ourselves and others.

Dictionaries define labyrinths as synonymous with mazes, filled with confusing and intricate passageways, but this is not accurate. Often confused with mazes, labyrinths are most frequently circular patterns leading to a central goal. Unlike a maze, you can't get lost in a labyrinth, and there are no decisions to make about which way to go.

The classic seven-circuit circular labyrinth has been in existence for at least four thousand years and is the most common type, but early Roman pavement labyrinths were usually square, and some cathedral labyrinths were octagonal.

Contrast such designs with progressive thinking, which utilizes maximum straight line efficiency and the shortest distance from here to there. Even our sense of time, history, and logic are linear. Conversely, the old expression "going around in circles" tends to convey that we are wasting time and/or are directionally challenged!

Despite these views, the labyrinth is purposefully the epitome of inefficiency because it has little to do with physically getting anywhere. Rather, it symbolically takes us away from our constant doing and into our "being," quieting our busy minds and allowing us to reconnect with neglected or forgotten parts of ourselves.

Walking these circles also takes us both outward and inward to regain balance in our lives. John Schneider, Ph.D., often had his clinical supervisees walk the Old Mission labyrinth adjacent to his office before they started their monthly review meetings. Under John's guidance, these individuals used three distinct reflective phases to re-center their broader clinical intentions:

> *Phase one—a time of release and quiet—shedding*
>
> *Phase two—a time to open and receive—focusing*
>
> *Phase three—a time to take what has been gained back out into the world— empowering*

Interestingly, the labyrinth has equal numbers of left and right turns with geometric regularity intended to balance both spheres of the brain. It is no coincidence that our own physical balancing mechanism utilizes a collection of semicircular canals in the middle ear also referred to as "the labyrinth."

Walking labyrinths potentially helps us restore our emotional and spiritual equilibrium. This is essential because nurses tend to exhibit an incredible generosity of self on behalf of others. However, we need paths that help keep us balanced with generosity to others and to ourselves while opening us to both give and receive love.

I believe there are two unspoken universal truths—we are born on an inhalation and a cry for love, and we die on an exhalation and a need for love. In his book *Anam Cara: A Book of Celtic Wisdom*, John O'Donahue, a renowned Irish poet and philosopher, says

Every human heart hungers for love. If you do not have the warmth of love in your heart, there is no real celebration and enjoyment. No matter how hard, competent, self-assured, or respected you are, no matter what you think of yourself or what others think of you, the one thing you deeply long for is love. No matter where we are, what we are, or what kind of journey we are on, we all need love. It is absolutely vital for a human life (8).

This poet also tells us that Celtic tradition uses light as a metaphor for the power and nurturing presence of love. Have you known and remembered people who seemed to shine an inner light just by their presence or their words? Children in particular have a wonderful way of being that innocent light.

I'm privileged to introduce each chapter of *The Ecology of Wellness for Nurses* with quotes or memories that reflect O'Donohue's theme of inner light and love. These have been submitted by nurses and nursing students as a source of renewal, sometimes over many years. I acknowledge their first names, titles, and years of nursing experience as validations that gently convey and uphold the worth of this profession while encouraging nurses every day in what they—what we—are about.

In Chapter One, I share the theoretical stepping stones of Milton Mayeroff, Sister Simone Roach, and Jean Watson. They have guided my philosophy of nursing practice for many years through literary contributions that both support wellness and strengthen my ecological perspective. Their validation of what is essential in work and life has molded the nurse I am today. Your own theoretical role models or nurse leaders whose voices resonate with the core of your nursing practice are important as well.

Chapter Two introduces another solid stepping stone that actually supports us throughout our life's journey both personally and professionally. This is the comprehensive transformative model of grief and loss envisioned, taught, and utilized by the clinical psychologist John Schneider. He poses three fundamental questions that all grieving human beings face: what is lost, what is left, and what is possible. His model also introduces the concept of validation as the door that opens us to genuine human to human relationships. To me, validation is the gossamer thread that quietly ties us heart to heart; it is one of the critical triad in healing presence.

In the same chapter, James E. Miller and Thomas R. Golden offer insightful guidance in their dual book *When a Man Faces Grief/A Man You Know Is Grieving*. As these titles reflect, nursing theory must be more comprehensively inclusive of men in all dimensions of caring, because the belief that women alone have the corner on compassion is simply inaccurate.

Chapter Three introduces the ecological model of wellness that asks us to evaluate the behavioral, constructed, and natural environments of our personal lives. These are crucial in guiding our wellness choices, actions, and feelings every moment of every day. Any change in one of these environments is integrally linked to the others in ways we may never have considered. Two types of change are reviewed as well as the concept of adaptation press.

Chapter Four carries us further into the deeper water of the ecological wellness model to focus on the spiritual space in which we explore the meaning of presence and healing presence to ourselves and others. In this spiritual space, our healing presence is most at home, guided by several key assumptions. Additionally, I define the triad of healing presence attributes as listening, validation, and hope.

In Chapter Five, I review the changes and challenges nursing is currently facing in a call for reformation in both nursing education and clinical preparation. Additionally, I discuss what I see as a renaissance in how and what nurses learn relative to their own wellness. Finally, I highlight forward strides whereby medical institutions are striving to reclaim the soul in healthcare and to restore compassionate caring for both employees and patients.

In Chapter Six, I highlight three transformative and compassionate paths that are gaining momentum and are already part of the renaissance in nursing. They are nurse coaching, a gender neutral nursing profession, and faith community nursing. Each is discussed and reframed within the ecological environments and relevancy to the spiritual space.

I close the book with Chapter Seven, in which I share my personal journey to embrace both the art and the heart of nursing over many years through the use of palliative music with my harp. I discuss the use of modes for healing and how an educational program first began with community volunteers, then grew to include hospital classes for hospital employees and/or hospice volunteers. I also highlight the support Munson Medical Center in Traverse City, Michigan, has provided in growing another healing modality for all its patients and staff.

Rachel Naomi Remen, M.D., writing in *My Grandfather's Blessings,* reminds us of what we are about through these words: "We do not serve the weak or broken. What we serve is the wholeness in each other and the wholeness in life. The part in you that I serve is the same part that is strengthened in me when I serve."

Together, let us continually seek the high-water mark of caring for both the reformation and renaissance that is not measured by our achievements but in the fullness of our healing presence. If reading this book compels one nurse to renew hope for our profession, that will be my blessing.

On Becoming a Nurse

*If there were ever a time to dare, to make a difference,
to embark on something new, it is now.*

Not necessarily for any grand cause,

*but for something that's your aspiration and your
inspiration.*

Something that tugs at your heart.

You owe it to yourself to make your days here count.

Begin

Goals worth achieving require tenacity.

*On the bad days there will be times when you want
to turn around, pack it up, call it quits. Walk away.*

But staying most affirms that you believe in yourself.

Courage always precedes the good days.

Persevere

With determination and the right skills,

You can do great things even in small ways.

Let your instincts, intellect, and inner wisdom

Guide your heart and hands.

Trust

Believe in the incredible power of—

> *Caring*
>
> *Humanity*
>
> *Working hard*

Laughing, hoping, dreaming, and

Doing something that makes a difference.

*Finally, let your presence always be remembered as a
reflection of*

one simple truth—   ***Love.***

SHARON OLSON, 1997, INSPIRED BY THE ANONYMOUS POEM "DREAM BIG"

As seen on a bumper sticker: "I am a nursing student. I am spending my life learning how to save your life." — Terri, R.N., 29 years

My mother Margaret Helen Mooney Sercu was a registered nurse and would have been eighty-nine years old in January, 2012. Her wisdom still guides me as I continue my own nursing journey. One of her memorable quotes was, "Don't be a nurse. It's slave labor, low pay, and you won't get any respect!" Mom was right of course. And so I have dedicated my nursing career to helping nursing become a safe and fair, well-paid, highly respected profession. More importantly, though, I have dedicated my life to being a strong, independent, and respectful person. Thanks, Mom! — MaryPat, R.N., M.S.N., 38 years

Dr. Ted Cline, a Traverse City surgeon who spoke at my nursing graduation ceremony, said, "One quality that will serve you and your patients the most is the importance of attention to detail." I have remembered it and lived by that my whole nursing career since 1970. Another quote by Jim Elliott I use is, "He is no fool who gives what he cannot keep to gain what he cannot lose." — Leone, R.N., 42 years

I have this quote by Florence Nightingale on my office wall: "Every year of her service a good nurse will say: I learn something every day." — Bonnie, R.N., 38 years

This quote is from George Washington Carver: "How far you go in life depends on your being tender with the young, compassionate with the aged, sympathetic with the striving and tolerant of the weak and strong. Because someday in your life you will have been all of these." — Leslie, R.N., B.S.N., 20 years

1

THREE ILLUMINATING GUIDES ON MY OWN NURSING JOURNEY

To speak with deeper wisdom—
To honor the whisper of your soul—
To love in all ways with a heart full of gratitude—
This is seeing with new eyes.

S. OLSON

Writing this chapter required me to collect, consolidate, and reflect on the influence of Milton Mayeroff, Sister Simone Roach, and Jean Watson, three theorists who have guided me professionally for almost half a century. It felt daunting and somewhat discouraging to presume I could put words to their influence. Where does one begin?

Whenever "writer's block" takes hold of me, I often retreat with a cup of tea in hand to where answers and life are most visible—our peaceful sunroom. This place of light and nature surrounds us to the east, south, and west. It is to the south that I nurture the perennial gardens that emerge and offer their cycles of beauty year after year. It was to the south that an idea was offered as I gazed on the snow-covered garden.

These authors, I realized, comprise my own perennial garden of knowing. Their predictability in all types of professional weather steadfastly assures their continued blooming. In the 1970s, it was the philosopher Milton Mayeroff who began pollinating and then fertilizing the seeds of caring as a central role in the lives of nurses and, in particular, in my life as a nurse.

As I briefly reflect on the contributions these theorists have made to my growth as a nurse, I humbly encourage you to consider whom it is that you have planted in your garden of knowing.

MILTON MAYEROFF

To help another person grow is at least to help him to care for something or someone apart from himself, and it involves encouraging and assisting him to find and create areas of his own in which he is able to care. Also it is to help that other person to come to care for himself by becoming responsive to his own need to care to become responsible for his own life.

MILTON MAYEROFF, *ON CARING*

I have a very used and cherished book by the late Milton Mayeroff (1925–1979) entitled *On Caring*. First published in 1971, it cost ninety-five cents yet still remains priceless to me. In just one hundred pages, his words capture both the fullness and the essence of caring and being cared for.

Mayeroff believed caring involves devotion, trust, patience, humility, honesty, knowing the other, respecting the primacy of the process, hope, and courage. Although he doesn't explicitly use the word "love," it is easy to discern these attributes as facets of the same diamond.

Also, he stressed that caring is primarily a process and not a series of goal-oriented services. Caring is not always agreeable, it is sometimes frustrating, and it is seldom easy. Yet while caring holds both pain and joy, it also profoundly helps us discover the fullness and meaning of life.

In 1995, Warren Reich wrote a classic article titled "History of the Notion of Care." His summary of Mayeroff's work described a "personalist vision" that takes the idea of care in a new and personal direction with the purpose of helping us understand and integrate our own lives more effectively. This vision encourages both a narrow and wide framework of connection with individuals sensing "from the inside" what the other person or self needs in order to grow in his or her own right (12).

Mayeroff's vision also resonated with Madeleine Leininger, the founder of transcultural caring, who emphasized the necessity of a "world view" that seeks a broader gestalt of another person's lifeways and cultural perspectives (*Caring—An Essential Human Need*, 5).

KNOWING

From Mayeroff's perspective, our failure to realize how much knowing there is in caring emanates from our propensity to restrict knowledge arbitrarily to what can be verbalized. He explained that caring knowledge includes the following interrelated perspectives:

- *Explicit knowing*—our ability to tell what we know and put it into words
- *Implicit knowing*—the how we know, which is difficult to articulate
- *Direct knowing*—information that is personally validated
- *Indirect knowing*—information that is "second-hand" (15)

Barbara Carper expanded this concept of knowing when she published her doctoral research on four fundamental patterns of knowing in nursing, stressing that none of the patterns alone is sufficient or mutually exclusive. She defined the four patterns as:

- *Empirical*—factual, descriptive information ultimately aimed at developing generalizable abstract and theoretical explanations.
- *Esthetics*—the empathic quality and openness of nurses to experience another's feelings as their own. Also, this pattern captures the art of individual nursing talents expressed through creativity in balance, rhythm, and harmony with the whole of caring.
- *Personal*—considered by Carper to be the most difficult pattern to master and to teach while also being the most essential to understanding the meaning of individual health and well-being. This pattern is tantamount to knowing and actualizing our individual self in relation to another human being, a relationship that reflects the reciprocity of interpersonal contacts that influence a person not only becoming

ill but also coping with illness and hopefully becoming well.

- ◆ *Ethical*—focused on matters of obligation or what "ought" to be done. More than simply knowing the norms or ethical codes, this pattern is also subject to including judgments of moral value in relation to motives, intentions, and traits of character. Both goals and actions involve choices made, in part, on the basis of these judgments that occasionally may also be in conflict (15–21).

In Chapter Five, I will again revisit knowing as transformed understanding and truth according to Dr. Parker Palmer.

M. Simone Roach

*The human person is not a problem to be solved,
but a mystery to be contemplated.*

**M. Simone Roach, *Caring from the Heart:
The Convergence of Caring and Spirituality***

Sister Simone Roach's contributions as a nursing educator have profoundly influenced and reinforced the central purpose of nursing as caring in both the United States and Canada for many years.

In 2010, as a retired nursing professor, she was appointed a member of the Order of Canada for her contributions as a leader in nursing education and for establishing the first code of ethics for nurses in Canada. Her book *The Human Act of Caring* offers the following quote as both an inspiration and an imperative for caring human relationships that is not intended to be exclusively for those whose lives are inspired by an expressed religious faith:

Love is patient, love is kind. It does not envy, it does not boast, it is not proud. It is not rude, it is not self-seeking, it is not easily angered, it keeps no recovery of wrongs. Love does not delight in evil but rejoices with truth. It always protects, always trusts, always hopes, always perseveres. Love never fails (1 Cor. 13. 4–8, New International Version).

Another theological perspective of caring as a basis for building community reported by Thomas Dubay in his book *Caring: A Biblical Theology of Community* uses the word "caring" as synonymous with love. He expresses it this way:

One loves when one cares and it reflects a genuine concern for the good of the other aside from what one may derive for oneself. Love and caring are primal. Loving is caring, deep love is deep caring; passionate love is passionate caring…It is to become the other in mind and heart, to love the other's interests. To care is to become one's brother, one's sister (23).

ATTRIBUTES OF CARING

Of continuing relevance today in our nursing practice are Simone Roach's five essential caring attributes (she refers to these as "the 5 C's") that evolved over time in response to two questions: What specific behaviors are evident when the nurse is caring, and which specific caring behaviors are essential for nursing practice? She notes that while not mutually exclusive, they serve as a helpful basis for specific caring behaviors and are not presented as an exhaustive list. The 5 C's encompass:

- *Confidence*—belief not only in ourselves but rather in what we have to offer in a trusting and authentic professional relationship. We must come to the bedside with confidence in the belief that our genuine presence has the potential to foster connectedness for mutual respect, truth, and trust.

♦ *Conscience*—moral awareness that directs our behavior according to our belief systems. This awareness values self and others. While sometimes referred to as "a call to care," it reflects a compass that directs our lives as a foundational moral experience.

♦ *Compassion*—indispensable to the caring relationship, presupposing and operating from a competence appropriate to the demands of human care. As a way of living, compassion embodies an awareness of one's relationship with all living creatures, engenders a response of participation in the experience of another, evokes a sensitivity to the pain and brokenness of the other, and upholds a quality of presence that allows one to share with and make room for the other. Compassion without competence may be no more than a meaningless, if not harmful, intrusion into the life of a person or persons needing help.

♦ *Competence*—having the knowledge, judgment, skills, energy, motivation, and experience required to respond appropriately to another human being on behalf of our profession, with the recognition that competence without compassion can be brutal and inhumane.

♦ *Commitment*—complex affective response characterized by a convergence between one's desires and one's obligation and by a deliberate choice to act in accordance with them. It is also an investment of self in a task, a person, or choice that becomes so internalized as a value that it is not considered a burden (58–65).

She summarizes the 5 C's this way:

[The 5 C's] were used as a broad framework suggesting categories of human behavior within which professional caring may be expressed. In compassionate and competent acts; in relationships qualified by confidence; through informed sensitive conscience; and through commitment and fidelity, specific manifestations of caring are actualized. Explicitly identifying such caring acts remains a task for the future (67).

In working with students learning modal music for healing, I have added one more C—Courage. As Amy Colombo notes in "Opening, Listening, and Caring through the Strings of a Harp," courage is also necessary as "volunteers bravely and willingly share music with an openness and flexibility to accept whatever the outcome" (*Your Gift*, 130).

Ultimately, to speak and live one's truth requires courage. I write informed by my insights, past experiences, sensitivity to the present, and a vision for what is yet possible. There is always something more for nurses to learn about ourselves from patients. They are most remarkable teachers.

In *Caring from the Heart: The Convergence of Caring and Spirituality*, Simone Roach notes that the heart is the primary organ of one's being and the center of life, embracing the core of each person's response to being human. Caring is profoundly:

♥ Revealed in uniquely established patterns of different cultures

♥ Manifested by all who share a common human journey

- ♥ Expressed in heroic ways
- ♥ Made visible in relationships
- ♥ Known through the spiritual nourishment of aesthetic experience
- ♥ Expressed and made visible through music and art
- ♥ Illuminated in an educational environment in which a human caring model is primary
- ♥ Taught in response to a hunger for spirituality in the educational aspirations of students and faculty alike (5)

She also acknowledges her concern regarding evolving professional challenges:

> People in organized human services everywhere are experiencing the pressures of downsizing, of major structural changes, of alternating corporate styles, of radical shifts in management in response to financial deficits and government priorities. In the face of these pressures, it is more important than ever that we not lose sight of the core of human service, that we not fall into the trap of economic and technological expediency (6).

These words were written fifteen years ago, yet visionaries have a way of seeing what we cannot yet see for ourselves. This is also true of Jean Watson.

JEAN WATSON

Caring begins with being present, open to compassion, mercy, gentleness, loving-kindness, and equanimity toward and with self before one can offer compassionate caring to others—actively, joyfully participating in all of it, the pain, the joy, the everything.

JEAN WATSON, *NURSING: THE PHILOSOPHY AND SCIENCE OF CARING*

In *Nursing: The Philosophy and Science of Caring*, Jean Watson reminds us that caring science embraces all ways of knowing/being/doing: ethical, intuitive, personal, empirical, aesthetic, and even spiritual/metaphysical ways of knowing and being (18). Her continually evolving work and theoretical development has dramatically enriched nursing practice. She has guided us with her carative factors from 1979 into the future with what she now refers to as Caritas Processes. Jean intentionally uses the word *caritas* as derived from the Latin meaning "to cherish, to appreciate, to give special, if not loving, attention to" as an explicit connection between caring and love (39).

Brief highlights of the ten Caritas Processes are:

+ Practicing loving-kindness and equanimity for self and others
+ Being authentically present
+ Cultivating one's own spiritual practices and deepening self-awareness
+ Developing and sustaining a helping/trusting, authentic caring relationship
+ Being present to and supportive of the expression of positive and negative feelings as a connection with deeper spirit of self and the one being cared for
+ Creative use of self and all ways of knowing/being/doing as part of the caring process

- Engaging in genuine teaching/learning experiences within the context of caring relationships attending to the whole person while attempting to stay within the other's frame of reference (i.e., evolving to a "coaching" role versus a more conventional imparting of information)
- Creating a healing environment at all levels
- Reverently and respectfully assisting with basic needs: holding an intentional, caring consciousness of touching and working with the embodied spirit of another, honoring unity of being, and allowing for a spirit-filled connection
- Opening and attending to spiritual, mysterious, unknown existential dimensions of life/death/ suffering and, in so doing, "allowing for a miracle" (31)

A summary of Caritas literacy (this word is used instead of the technical term "competencies") can be found in Addendum III of *Nursing: The Philosophy and Science of Caring*. See also additional website resources at the end of this chapter.

Conclusion

Milton Mayeroff, Simone Roach, and Jean Watson have had "staying power" with me because they express philosophies that resonate and encourage a new ecological dialogue for wellness that must be planted upstream for a future generation of nurses. If we can embrace this wellness approach, I am convinced it will uphold nurses in the worst of times and, more importantly, validate them in the very best of nursing practices *over* time.

References

Dubay, T. 1973. *Caring: A Biblical Theology of Community.* Denville, NJ: Dimension Books.

Carper, B. Oct., 1978. "Fundamental Patterns of Knowing in Nursing." *Advances in Nursing Science* 1(1): 13–23.

Colombo, A. 2012. *Your Gift: An Educational, Spiritual, and Personal Resource for Hospice Volunteers.* Sharon Olson, ed. 122–135. Traverse City, MI: Seasons Press.

Leininger, M., ed. 1981. *Caring—An Essential Human Need.* Detroit: Wayne State University Press.

Mayeroff, M. 1971. *On Caring.* New York: Harper & Row.

Reich, W., ed. 1995. "History of the Notion of Care." *Encyclopedia of Bioethics.* Revised edition. Five volumes. New York: Simon & Schuster Macmillan. 319–331.

Roach, M. S., ed. 1997. *Caring from the Heart: The Convergence of Caring and Spirituality.* New Jersey: Paulist Press.

Roach, M. S. 1992. *The Human Act of Caring.* Ottawa, Ontario: Canadian Hospital Association Press.

Watson J. 2008. *Nursing: The Philosophy and Science of Caring.* Revised edition. Boulder, Co: The University Press of Colorado.

ADDITIONAL RESOURCES

Watson Caring Science Institute International Caritas
Consortium. www.watsoncaringscience.org.

International Association of Human Caring. www.human-
caring.org.

The Future of Nursing—Leading Change, Advancing Health. 2011.
Committee on the Robert Wood Johnson Foundation
Initiative on the future of nursing at the Institue of
Medicine. http://www.nap.edu/catalog/12956.html.

I am a single mom of three and work full time. This quote by Franki Dubin is posted above my desk to remind me that even though my heart's desire to be a nurse is on temporary hold, I will reach that goal as long as I keep my eyes on the prize. "Do not settle for less than exactly what you want. Your heart's desires are there for a reason. Chase them. Pursue them relentlessly. Do not lose sight of your goals. They are your very reason for being." — Kim, nursing student

I was "called" to nursing at an early age when I assisted my Cherokee grandmother (who was the regional midwife and veterinarian) in delivering calves, piglets, and foals and also treating their various ailments. My career has been very fulfilling and diverse in various areas of caring. The highlight was my participation in the advent of hospice care in the 1980s, and I was also privileged to witness President Ronald Reagan sign the Medicare Hospice Coverage document. I entered nursing school when I was thirty-three, and now at seventy-eight I continue to be involved in nursing. — Lee, R.N., M.S.N., L.M.T., 45 years

I recall one of those learning days we all have as we grow up in this work. I was about thirty then—eight years as a nurse working in oncology, night shift on the weekends. The whole story is not so important. What my head nurse did was line up behind me in a confrontation with a doc who didn't know me and was upset by something he thought I didn't do. I was off duty so he sounded off to her. She told him, "That doesn't make sense to me; this is a very reliable nurse." Simple enough. It changed the nature of the equation. And I never forgot it. She could have thrown me under the bus but instead she gave me a lasting piece of my self-image. We should all be so with our fellow nurses. — Anne, R.N., F.N.P., 34 years

2

SEEING DEEP AND WIDE—
VALIDATING OUR LOSSES
AND GRIEF'S JOURNEY

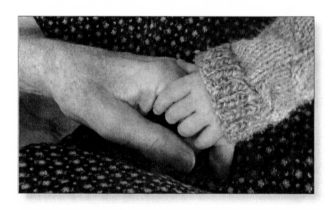

In the solitude of the heart we can truly listen to the pains of the world because there we can recognize them not as strange and unfamiliar pains, but as pains that are indeed our own. There we can see that what is most universal is most personal.

HENRI NOUWEN, *REACHING OUT*

One cannot begin to understand the broad concept of true wellness without first understanding the profound influence that losses and grief have in both molding and changing the course of our lives.

This chapter presents two important concepts. First, our capacity as nurses to walk a healing journey is in large measure related to the validation we have received from others and what we are able to give ourselves. It begins with our personal stories, because the more we are validated, the more we are able to validate others. Validation is also incredibly important to every nurse in the triad of healing presence discussed in Chapter Four.

Second, validation is integral to grief's transformative model that John Schneider, a clinical psychologist, presents in *Finding My Way—From Trauma to Transformation: The Journey through Loss and Grief.* He defines grieving as "a process of discovering the extent to and the limits of what is lost, what is left, and what is possible" (104). He also reminds us that knowing something about grief does not hasten the process or lessen its pain. However, such knowledge can reassure us that we are not alone on our journey. We see with new eyes when the door of our soul must open to grief because this journey is really about self-discovery.

With appropriate support and validation, the health-seeking part of us wants to discover what it is we have lost and what remains afterward so that we can know what to do with it in the context of the wholeness of our lives. Surprisingly, our deep grief can be creative, compelling us to write poetry or stories or to draw, paint, weave, or complete artistic projects we had set aside. This is grief's voice calling us to open our deeper self to another way of healing and to express our private deep sorrow.

Perhaps you might wonder why a chapter on validation is necessary for nurses. It is necessary because every time we approach a patient's bedside or sit next to a patient in a clinical setting gathering information, the story we hear will be inexplicably wrapped with some measure of change, loss, and grief. Inside, each patient holds a story, and each patient yearns for someone who cares enough to listen. In those moments, our caring will be remembered not by what we do but by how we make our patients feel when we validate their losses and grief journey in all its fullness.

A self-validation awareness reflection is therefore included at the end of this chapter for your personal contemplation.

VALIDATION, "A KEY TO THE DOOR OF HEALING"

What does the word "validation" really mean? It derives from the Latin word *valere* meaning to "be strong" and is defined by Webster's College Dictionary as "a confirmation, or substantiation of something or someone." As a verb, it means "to confirm or establish the truthfulness or soundness of something."

In 1989, my husband John and I were discussing the attributes of caring at a restaurant when we began focusing our thoughts on validation. A rich framework began to take shape as we enthusiastically scribbled our ideas on numerous paper napkins. I wish I had kept those napkins as a reminder of what evolved to the following refined definition:

Validation: a holistic, positive and genuine, nonjudgmental encounter that communicates a commitment to the best (or highest) self, that appreciates the moment and the journey, that provides witness, gentle honesty, and suspends judgment (Schneider 350)

To validate someone does not necessarily require a verbal exchange. It may be a gentle touch or a glance of admiration, love, compassion, or knowing. It is more than the "verbal M&M's" of compliments or simple recognition that tends to be short-lived in our memories. Instead, true validations like the one below are remembered over time because they resonate with that "best self" within each of us (Olson and Schneider 27).

> *When the nurse first entered my husband's ICU room, he introduced himself and said, "You know, I have two patients in this room—you and your husband." He held true to those words to the very end, and I will never forget his validation of my needs as well.*

People we remember fondly in some way, shape, or form validated us by words, deeds, or simply by their quiet presence when we needed it most. It is said, "We cannot give what we have not received," and so it is with validation. In order to be able to validate others, it must begin with ourselves. The simple truth is that the more we are validated, the more we are capable of validating those around us. Our own self-validations both affirm and nourish the best self within us to mindfully "walk our talk." After all, we never know when small acts of healing presence, caring, and kindness will quietly touch another's life story. Further, on a personal level, we never know when we will be surprised by joy.

I was recently approached in the grocery store by a woman I didn't recognize. She simply wanted to remind me that I was one of the harpers who had played at the bedside for her loved one at a difficult time in the hospital and to express how much the music had meant. This is a lovely example of how a validation I had offered came full circle to validate me.

Paradoxically, it is the ones we love the most whom we tend to validate the least. Why is this? Most often, we assume they already know how we feel about them. In the meantime, we lose precious opportunities to validate their worth and meaning in our lives, all the while knowing full well that the more they are validated, the more they learn to reciprocate kindness and caring.

Validation is communication in its fullest sense guided by five principles, all of which must be evident. They are:

- *Putting aside judgment.* A basic tenet is that nonjudgmental moments convey safety and positive regard while also encouraging opportunities for self-discovery and safety.

- *Committing to the best self.* This means holding hope for something not visible or tangible at the moment. It includes belief in a person's capacity to rise to the occasion when obstacles seem impossible. From inner strength and with time, the best self is transformed to more than it was before, despite having less.

- *Appreciating both the moment and the journey.* This requires acknowledging the significance of past, present, and future. It means staying in the moment as long as it needs to be to allow appreciation both of the fullness of the moment and the significance of the journey.

- *Witnessing both the moment and the journey.* This is "being there" and being fully present. It poignantly writes both a history and a story into our remembrance.

- *Being honest and gentle.* Honesty is the process of acknowledging reality and the fullness of the here and now. No matter how powerful the truth, we trust that we have within us the ability to gently embrace our integrity.

Using these principles, validation is therapeutic because it acknowledges the human condition, whatever that may be. It affirms strengths and encourages self-care. It can also challenge people to renew relationships that may have been strained and to forgive misunderstandings. Overall, its therapeutic value comes in providing safety, nurturance, and hope for the health and well-being of self and relationships. It also supports the belief that individuals' and patients' attempts at coping represent their best efforts in the *present moment*, at this point in their journey.

The Importance of Validating the Masculine Style of Grieving

In their dual book *When a Man Faces Grief* and *A Man You Know Is Grieving*, Thomas Golden and James Miller share their collective wisdom from personal grief experiences and also as professionals who work with grieving men. They suggest that in our culture a feminine style is well known and characterized by emphasizing interactions with others, expressing the emotions—often tearfully—and communicating verbally the loss's impact as well as reflecting on the past.

For men, they note, our culture has created an idealized image of strength, confidence, and independence. Concomitantly, in grief, men are discouraged from openly expressing their sadness and are encouraged "to forge ahead," doing whatever the circumstances call for (Miller and Golden 12). Not surprisingly, this idealized image of grief has been shaped and reinforced by all types of media, movies, and television sitcoms.

It is important to remember that a masculine style of grief may be used by women just as a feminine style may surface at times in a man's grief journey. All these styles of grieving must be validated. Specifically, it is important to remember that individuals grieving in a masculine style will often:

- Grieve in their own way, influenced by who they are, what they've experienced, and how they've been raised
- Use fewer words than those around them
- Be inclined to use their strengths to connect with and heal their pains
- Choose to tap into their grief by taking action more than through interaction
- Place value on independence, quiet, and solitude as they grieve
- Find meaning in caring for those around them as one aspect of the grieving process
- Wish to honor their loss through action that impacts the future more than talking about the past
- Use their courage to stand in the tension of grief with all its turbulence, loneliness, and unpredicability
- Build on their grief experience and use it for their own growth (Golden and Miller 32)

However grief manifests itself, it leads both men and women from the security of what used to be toward the possibility of what can yet be. It doesn't fill up the holes; it leads to greater wholeness. Grief doesn't smooth over what happened; it exposes loss to the light so it can be dealt with and worked through as much and as fully as possible. And, grief doesn't lead people back to their former lives. It leads them forward to new or renewed lives. It doesn't patch things together; it helps bring healing (Miller and Golden 31).

THE COMPLEXITIES OF LOSS

Each of us experiences a life-long process of responding to change and loss. Every change, major or minor, ripples through our lives and sometimes feels as powerful as a tidal wave wreaking havoc on the most fortified individuals and families. Even when these waters recede, there is still much more to grief than what happens in the first few days or months.

While reading the following sections, consider the times when you have experienced significant losses and either put your grief "on hold" or began immediately to deal with the consequences. Perhaps there was a time when you were deep in your own grief yet still had to work a twelve-hour shift or see patients in your clinic. The breadth of loss is both deep and wide, is not always connected with death, and at times may not even be evident to others who know you well. Consider the following examples of loss:

- Loss of innocence and assumptions
- Loss of identity, such as happens with retirement, divorce, or widowhood
- Loss of sense of self and perhaps of soul tied to a role and the decisions we make
- Transgenerational loss
- Circumstantial or significant material losses, including natural disasters
- Shared losses
- Disenfranchised losses representing violence/abuse/violations of a person's spirit or soul (Schneider 18–24)

You may have your own personal example that is not listed. Regardless of the source, there is a journey we all travel at our own pace and in our own time. Ultimately, we face three challenges that tend to come in sequence for most people in normal grieving before the transformative potential in grief can be realized. These challenges are finding what's lost, what remains, and what's possible.

In his comprehensive review of the grief journey, John Schneider notes that every phase of grief has behavioral, cognitive, emotional, physical, and spiritual aspects. For a thorough narrative of each of these aspects, please reference *Finding My Way—From Trauma to Transformation: The Journey through Loss and Grief.*

The First Challenge: Discovering What and How Much Has Been Lost

What one beholds of grief is the least part of it.
ANONYMOUS

The beginning of grief is a time of great vulnerability and of necessity entails active grieving. This is an important part of discovering what and how much has been lost and includes two important components. One involves the coping strategies of either holding on to the loss or letting it go. Similar to the "fight or flight syndrome," coping strategies reflect our biological mechanism for responding to threat.

Coping by Holding On. When we fight or hold on to loss, we are trying to overcome what threatens us. We won't give in to the loss or give up. We're determined not to relinquish what's meaningful. For example, some patients will tenaciously cling to life until their child graduates or the holidays are over.

Holding on isn't always positive. It can be exhausting holding on to our denial of what's ahead. We can even be tempted to avoid the loss. For example, we may not want to see loved ones when they are very ill or dying because we want to hold the image of the person as healthy. Later, however, we may regret that we were not witness to their illness or dying process.

Coping by Letting Go. As part of the natural ebb and flow of coping with the beginning of grief, letting go balances holding on. One uses energy; the other conserves it. One is overly optimistic; the other is excessively pessimistic. One romanticizes the best self; the other denies its existence. Between them, they maximize our capacity to grieve while continuing to survive. Letting go is essentially a flight from the reality of the loss, and when used to the extreme, it doesn't really address the loss. This in turn poses a risk of stopping the grieving process altogether (Schneider 182). Eventually, we do begin to grasp the full extent of what we've lost, and coping by holding on or letting go becomes less a part of the grieving process.

The other aspect of active grieving is awareness. This is the most critical phase of grief and can be the most painful, lonely, helpless, and hopeless of times anyone faces. This is the place beneath the surface where we cannot breathe. There is no fight or flight here, only numbing stillness. There is no light, only darkness—*and that is as it should be* (Schneider 198).

Entering Deep Awareness. Previously we were unable to admit the depth of the loss in the two coping strategies of holding on and letting go, but now we enter a time of deep recognition that:

- Measures the full extent of what is missing and crowds out everything else
- Reveals what can never be again
- Is a crisis of being—we can't return to a time before the loss occurred but neither are we

ready to move forward to a time when the loss
can be integrated

- Makes it impossible to be in awareness without
  it being a total experience
- Forces us to experience sadness, pain, and emp-
  tiness on many levels, with the original loss
  only one aspect of the larger whole that must
  be explored
- Is unpredictable and can be triggered by a
  memory, a song, a place, an anniversary, or a
  season
- Imbues a sense of fragility to our whole being

One of the mysterious transformations of grief is the capacity,
in the absolute depths of awareness, to find a connection that
makes it possible to go on. We gain courage by grieving so we
can do what we need to do. We find strength we didn't know
we had because we must. We face limits and find new options
because we have no choice. One woman described finding her
courage and strength this way:

*Over the course of four weeks in ICU, I watched my husband
slowly continue to deteriorate from one medical complica-
tion after another, eventually becoming unresponsive. One
evening, very exhausted, I went home for a few hours of sleep.
Suddenly, at 3:00 a.m., I awakened knowing with full clarity
exactly what Jim wanted me to do. I called his ICU nurse and
told him I wanted to bring my husband home with hospice
care as soon as possible. By early morning, the order was
written for transfer to hospice services, and Jim was home
by late afternoon. I still think about that early morning decision. You see, I had to let go of my denial and hear my very
own words acknowledge with total awareness for the very*

*first time that my beloved husband was dying. It took more
courage than I knew I had to accept that devastating reality.*

THE SECOND CHALLENGE:
DISCOVERING WHAT REMAINS
AS WE INTEGRATE OUR LOSSES
AND MOVE ON

The lowest ebb is the turn of the tide.
HENRY WADSWORTH LONGFELLOW

Eventually, the time comes when grief no longer feels like a
crushing burden. For so long, awareness of the loss was the
core of our consciousness. There was no getting away from
it, except for very brief respites. There are still times when we
slip back into awareness, but these times aren't so frightening
and the loss no longer consumes every waking moment. This
doesn't mean that if new information surfaces on the loss that
we won't return to awareness with its all-consuming qualities.
Again, we stay with it as long as it takes to evaluate what has
been lost, given where we are at this time. The following comments reflect this vacillating discovery process:

- ◆ "Some days I can't seem to hit a predictable
  stride emotionally, much less a step forward
  with any confidence."
- ◆ "Just when I think I'm on solid ground, I step
  into another grief sinkhole."
- ◆ "What good is a full tank of gas when you've
  lost your road map of life? I still don't know
  where the hell I'm headed, but I keep driving!"

The transition from the discovery of what is lost to the discovery of what remains is perhaps the most critical threshold

one can cross in the grief process. When it occurs, we experience the peace of accepting a loss for what it is. Searching ends. Energy is conserved. Healing germinates (Schneider 222). This is also the point at which many caregiving systems complete their commitments of support. But while all this may be true, it doesn't mean that grieving is complete or that we don't need additional support.

Perspective...the Beginning of Healing. As awareness pangs ebb, we rest and heal the scars of what is missing. We stop trying to figure out the loss and let "soul healing" begin in its own quiet way. In solitude, we begin to sort out what remains, to find the remnants, and to restore what we can. Perhaps, for the first time in our lives, we allow self-compassion to gently help us put the lost pieces of our souls back where they belong, as the following stories reflect:

> *When our hospital went through a recent merger, a number of nursing positions were cut. I'd worked on a med-surg. unit for five years and loved what I did. I didn't expect to be "let go," but I was. It took me a year to find another job and heal from that experience and regain my professional confidence. I work at a specialty clinic now and it has turned out to be more rewarding than I ever thought possible. I never thought I would say this, but I don't think I'll ever go back to hospital nursing again.*

*   *   *

> *I have always believed there are no coincidences. The day my husband died was the same day my son and his wife found out that they were expecting a baby. That precious little girl was born on Christmas Day, giving me a gift beyond measure by revealing that there was something more beyond my grief that I could see, hold, and love.*

Perspective emerges because it involves acceptance. However, perspective is not the same as completion. Of necessity, perspective is a passive healing that calls us forward to fully know what is left. It takes time and patience to co-exist in peace with loss. Those who have healed from loss consistently identify several things that helped them:

- They had people who believed in them, who held their hope for them
- They hit bottom, often more than once
- They kept going long enough
- They rediscovered their best selves
- They felt safe to explore whatever they needed to about the loss

At this point, we are grieving something much larger that has to do with understanding human nature and the desire for wholeness. This wholeness requires fitting our loss into the very fabric of all our experiences in order to live fully. In other words, to begin living fully, we must integrate the loss with all its consequences (Schneider 237).

CROSSING THE THRESHOLD— INTEGRATING, RE-SOLVING AND RESTORING

When you walk to the edge of all the light you have and take that first step into the darkness of the unknown, you must believe that one of two things will happen: there will be something solid for you to stand upon, or you will be taught how to fly.

PATRICK OVERTON, "FAITH"©

The above inspiring words keenly express what happens when we "cross the threshold" and begin integrating, re-solving, and restoring after loss.

Integrating. Integrating our loss exists on the cusp between what's left and what's possible. We are often able to see ahead long before it becomes a reality. It takes courage to integrate loss because we face fear, heartache, and many other emotions in addition to hard work still ahead. We must define new routines, new disciplines, and new commitments, especially to self-care, in order to be more psychologically hardy and ready for what's coming.

Re-solving. "Re-solve" as it is intended here is not the same as resolution, which implies that we can somehow "finish" the loss, put it away, and never explore it again. However, John Schnieder uses this term to mean determination to go on *because* of rather than in *spite* of a loss. He means "having resolve" rather than "being resolved." Literally, to re-solve is to solve the loss again from a new vantage point, exploring all the aspects to discover a new way of living, and integrating what we have lost into the future (245).

Restoring. By integrating the loss, we also accept the impossibility of retrieving the form of what we've lost. However, the essence of what we had remains. Our ability to still feel the warmth, inspiration, love, and what uniquely characterized the relationship validates the essence of what has been lost. Indeed, our grief journey has brought us to the doorstep of a profound paradox: "We are more than we were before, despite having less."

Schneider refers to this as the existential moment when we decide whether we can and will step across the threshold of "how it was" to "what will be" and validate our personal responsibility for who we now are and what we are to do with our future. He calls this a holistic reformation or restoration of our best self, and when it occurs, we won't and literally can't go back to who we were. Examples of statements that reflect the integration of what loss has taught us thus far include:

- "I know deep inside that I've changed."
- "I see with new eyes."
- "I feel more connected to the world and nature."
- "I feel more of a connection to humanity as a whole."
- "I think more deeply about my life's direction and future choices."
- "I have a deeper appreciation of what is really important in life, love, friendships, and family."
- "I've challenged and altered some of my long-standing assumptions and beliefs."

Thus far, grief has consisted of

- *Coping:* actively grieving the way things were and can no longer be
- *Awareness:* relinquishing the form of connections and discovering the internal capacities to go on in order to retain the essence of those connections
- *Perspective:* experiencing the healing that comes from discovering the capacity to tolerate hopelessness, helplessness, despair, pain, uncertainty, loneliness, and the absence of love's expression and reception gracefully, with courage, remorse, empathy, and forgiveness
- *Integration:* integrating mind, body, and spirit to resolve, remember, restore, or make right the consequences of loss

Yet what lies ahead is finding our capacity to create significance in life where it has been absent. All we have for this journey is hope—hope for a mending of what we've lost and for a new vitality. By reformulating and transforming our loss, we can now begin to live that hope, or return to it more quickly.

The Third Challenge: Finding What's Possible and Reformulating Our Losses

Do you think that death will somehow fail to catch us all, no matter what we are doing?...What do you want to be doing when it catches you?...If you have anything you believe is more important to have done or be doing when death comes, get to work on that.
Epictetus, Greek Stoic philosopher (55–135 CE)

There does come a time in the grieving process when life looks very different, when opportunities now exist *because* of the loss rather than in *spite* of it. "Reformulating" literally means "to re-form," to build something new. We affirm what matters—the basic nature of affections, affiliations, and values. We would not have grown or found so much meaning and purpose in life had the loss not happened the way it did. We also stop trying to go back to the old self because there is a provocative reality that what we need to be about now cannot wait.

I read an article recently about Michael J. Fox who founded the Michael J. Fox Foundation for Parkinson's Research (MJFF) to help usher in a new future for people with Parkinson's disease—a future filled with hope. He said, "It's ironic that I had to quit my day job to do my life's work" (Gora 15).

This quote struck a very personal chord with me because after my husband's death, I did in fact quit my "day job" to move in a new professional direction. I am not implying or even advocating that people who experience a significant loss should quit their jobs. Rather, it is as if each of us in our own time and way comes to see and understand what is really important in both our personal and professional lives. I finally listened to what my best self had been whispering to me for many years. You could say that I am now embarking on a journey, moving out from the center of my own labyrinth to live more fully the significance of my life. The path seems familiar yet is profoundly different, and courage is my companion.

TRANSFORMATION— LIVING THE WHOLENESS OF LIFE

A number of years ago, we planted a tree in the center of our labyrinth honoring an amazing gentleman and the father of our dear friend Lee. In his nineties, he was still living a vibrant life until being admitted for a minor procedure in the same hospital Lee had worked at for many years as a nurse. A medical nursing error caused his death, and Lee suffered a difficult journey to healing on many levels both personally and professionally. She recently visited our home and spent healing time in the center of the labyrinth literally hugging the tree as a validation of the life, love, and grace her father represented. These attributes continue to be reflected as the essence of Lee's deep caring and love for her patients and family members.

The most important resource for personal growth in the face of losses lies in our capacity to understand the nature of the change we are experiencing. Once again, validation is essential for ourselves and for how the options we are considering affect us. If someone's choice comes from the best self, does it not need and deserve our wholehearted support (Schneider 299)?

Grief is the agent that empowers remarkable transformations that

- Emerge from the courage to face fully the consequences of change
- Result in the motivation to restore what can be restored
- Open the possibilities of new vistas and a more inclusive ability to love
- Restore self-confidence
- Free us to think about an ever-widening range of possibilities and choices
- Turn possibilities into probabilities and some dreams into realities
- Produce the autonomy that empowers the choices we eventually make
- Expand love and joy
- Shift us from a material or self-centered life to a more inclusive, altruistic, transpersonal one

CONCLUSION

There is no place where loss or growth potential does not exist. Nor is there any time when joy or sadness cannot appear. How fully can we nurses embrace life's defining moments with grace, acceptance, and gratitude through our own unique journeys? If we stay involved in living, we must also grieve losses, tragedies, traumas, and setbacks. Even our successes and the rewards that life provides hold aspects of grief. However, if we grieve with integrity when we must, we are then free to live fully the interludes in between. That is what transformation is all about. We find new strengths, a new unity of self, and new depths of love and caring that become gifts to ourselves and ultimately to our patients as we companion with them, however briefly, through their losses.

I close this chapter with a beautiful poem contributed by Anne Lanier, who spent twenty of her thirty-five years as an R.N. working as a hospice nurse.

PAIN AND BEAUTY

There are times when there are no words to express

The depth of pain in this world

Nor to express the beauty that is sometimes within pain

There was such a time when a child lay dying in his bed

His mother and his father were staying by his side

His mother sat silently holding his hand, stroking his arm

His father spoke softly, saying how proud they were of him, saying what a good boy he had been

The child, with eyes closed and before he died whispered back to them,

Because you were my mother

Because you were my father

ANNE LANIER, R.N.

Self-Validation Awareness Reflection

Complete the following statements. Which ones do you find most difficult to answer?

A person I remember who first validated me was:

I am most grateful for:

I savor:

My greatest joy:

My greatest strength:

My most significant limitation:

I am hard on myself for:

The hardest thing to accept:

I have forgiven:

I have not forgiven:

One of the most important ways I have changed:

I am most creative when:

(CONTINUED)

Self-Validation Awareness Reflection
(cont. from page 37)

I am at my best when:

My greatest loss:

I could not have made it this far without:

My greatest growth:

A recent positive change in my life has been:

My most important relationship:

My mission/calling in life:

If I were to receive "bad news" I would want to hear it from:

Finding My Way—From Trauma to Transformation: The Journey through Loss and Grief by John M. Schneider (revised with permission) © 2012

REFERENCES

Golden, T., and J. Miller. 1998. *When a Man Faces Grief.* Ft. Wayne, Indiana: Willowgreen Publishing.

Gora, S. Dec. 2011/Jan. 2012. "Outfoxing Parkinson's." *Neurology Now* 7(6): 14–19.

Miller, J., and T. Golden. 1998. *A Man You Know Is Grieving.* Ft. Wayne, Indiana: Willowgreen Publications.

Olson, S., and J. M. Schneider. Jan./Feb., 1990. "Validation: The Nature and Nurture of Validation." *New Realities* X(3): 25–28.

Schneider, J. M. 2012. *Finding My Way—From Trauma to Transformation: The Journey through Loss and Grief.* Traverse City, MI: Seasons Press.

Webster's College Dictionary. 1995. Costello, R., ed. New York: Random House.

When you are a nurse, you know that every day you will touch a life or a life touches yours. — Cheryl, R.N., 13 years

A little girl is standing on the beach throwing starfish that have been washed up onto the beach back into the ocean. When confronted by a man who said that her actions would make no difference because more and more starfish would keep washing onto the beach, she replied, "It makes a difference to this one!" as she threw it back into the sea. I always wear a starfish pin on my lab coat. I am privileged to care for elders, our most valuable natural resource. — Kathryn, G.N.P, 40 years

It's a good day at work when nobody dies and you didn't get yelled at. That way you can leave work with a positive feeling on most days. The other days will take care of themselves. — Michael, R.N., 27 years, the last 25 in adult critical care

This quote comes from Maggie Kuhn: "Old age is not a disease: it's not a social disaster; it's a gift of the Almighty." — Marsha, R.N., M.S.N., 40 years, geriatric specialty

My quote is from my mother Marjorie who was also a nurse since 1943 and joined the navy in 1944 as a nurse. She kept her license current until she was in her seventies. She was graceful in life and in death at the wonderful age of eighty-nine. Her quote is, "It is better to be kind than right." — Jane, R.N., 34 years

3

THE ECOLOGICAL MODEL OF WELLNESS

Perhaps it is the passion and commitment to the caring imperative in education and in health care that can shape the dialogue and the dialectic, frame the issues, and make a new clearing—a clearing whereby caring can be kept alive and space for new possibilities can emerge for teachers and students and systems alike.

JEAN WATSON, *THE CARING IMPERATIVE IN EDUCATION*

Sixteen years ago, half a world away, someone believed it was time to make a new clearing and space for new possibilities. In 1996, Alan Avery, a nurse and educator in the Department of Nursing and Midwifery at the University of New England, New South Wales, Australia, wrote an article entitled "Eco-Wellness Nursing: Getting Serious about Innovation and Change." In it, he called for a reformed nursing vision that would promote and empower people towards ecologically centered goals. He noted that

> Critical inquiry, context, action, discourse and reflection remain as important processes but require much broader and holistic insights, applications and horizons than previously accepted within nursing scholarship (70).

Calling for a different educational focus than currently existed, he suggested that

> The study of ecology, wellness, holism, and environmental practices that affect modern human ecoculture foster new models of adult learning/teaching. This enables students to become active, reflective, critical and creative learners distinct from the limiting and dependency-creating traditional pedagogical educational framework (72).

The article also provided examples of how an "eco-wellness" nurse might engage practically in terms of the caring process from an ecocentric health and wellness perspective.

I believe now more than ever that our profession must get serious about aggressively pursuing this agenda. Current local, national, and global environmental changes are affecting individuals and families in ways we never could have imagined. Therefore, I have bravely entered this relay for ecological wellness and willingly take up the baton from Avery to carry it a few more laps. I may not see the finish line in my lifetime, but every stride I make is worth it because this is the race our profession must win on behalf of our patients, families, and the environment.

In her book *My Grandfather's Blessings*, Rachel Naomi Ramen, M.D., said, "Sometimes if you stay the course long enough, divergent paths reveal themselves to have the same destination" (4). Despite my seemingly divergent higher education paths and nursing experiences over many years, I understand that my choices have always been framed by an ecological model. For example, in my continuing education with osteopathic courses as a nurse practitioner, I learned effective ways to treat musculoskeletal pain and restricted motion. Over more than ten years, one overarching premise guided my daily assessments: "Identify the pain; look elsewhere for the problem." Opening our lens of understanding to the "whole" of wellness requires just that —identifying the concerns and looking more broadly for the influences that might be possible to change.

In conversations today, there is increasing concern and dialogue encompassing the word "ecology." These conversations tend to be used in the context of assaults on or the preservation of our natural environment. However, more frequently, ecological discussions are now inclusive of the human element and the additional detrimental effects of the environment on individuals and families.

The word "ecology" derives from the Greek words *oikos* meaning "house" and *logos* meaning "word." While general knowledge may or may not cause change, ecological knowledge always inspires change at some level, even subtlety, because it holds personal meaning.

As early as 1978, Barbara Carper wrote about health being more than the absence of disease and how systems models explain a person's level of wellness at any particular point in time as a function of current and accumulated effects of interactions with their internal and external environments (14–15).

Subsequently, in 1979, Bubolz, Eicher, and Sontag envisioned three interrelated environments, the behavioral, the constructed, and the natural, representing what they called the "human ecological model." Every moment of every day, we are entwined with these environments to a greater or lesser degree, whether we are aware of it or not.

This chapter reviews two types of change—those both within and of individual, family, and work systems that may be pressed into adapting for change and/or survival. The behavioral, constructed, and natural environments are also presented. Invariably, we see things not as they are but as we are. Thus, I encourage you to thoughtfully reflect on the following two questions as you delve into each of the following environments:

Question one: What are the encouraging, life-empowering factors I see in this environment that support my wellness?

Question two: What are the discouraging, disempowering factors that impair my wellness?

An ecological wellness survey is included at the end of this chapter. It is intended to help you consider what encouraging as well as discouraging influences are occurring within your personal environments, what adaptation presses exist, and if you were to consider a wellness change, what environment you might start with.

CHANGE AND ADAPTATION PRESS

From a systems perspective, Watzlawick et al. noted two types of change that our lives may be touched by. First order change is change that occurs within a family system such as when a child leaves home to attend college or perhaps a family member has surgery and requires a period of rehabilitation. The adjustments families must make in these scenarios are usually not without some challenges, but ultimately the system holds together (10).

By contrast, second order change is a change of the system. Here, everything changes! Losing a job, a home, or experiencing divorce or a death within the family system falls under second order change, as does having a child. Such situations demand reorganization around an entirely new premise and disrupt all semblance of order in our lives (11).

Ultimately, second order change introduces a complex milieu of needs, including the need to understand the breadth and depth of our losses which may be profound or subtle. Regardless, our grief response involves resolving the questions of what remains, what can be restored, and what is still possible. How we adapt is a journey uniquely our own.

In 1988, my research with Michigan hospice programs included identifying factors that encouraged change through their organizations' stages of development. Within each of the four stages, described as stage one: organizing; stage two: formalizing; stage three: consolidating; and stage four; extending, the concept of adaptation was seen as a central challenge as the hospices grew in staff, volunteers, and service area (41–47).

I defined adaptation at that time as the process of responding to environmental demands (stressors) while enabling hospice programs to maintain a steady state. Coincidentally, the research demonstrated another reality that led me to further refine this definition to include "adaptation press," which relates to the environmental demands that are exerted upon a system that may encourage and/or force adaptation regardless of an otherwise steady state (40).

Increasingly, change is a personal or professional "ultimatum" with very few options. The challenge is, how do we respond to that pressure to adapt and still retain our integrity and priorities within each of the following unique environments? In other words, how do we nurture wellness ecologically in the behavioral, constructed, and natural environments in which we live and work?

THE BEHAVIORAL ENVIRONMENT

Our behavioral environment is the broad sweep of our psycho/social, spiritual, and emotional histories that have formed our thoughts, emotional responses, values, and beliefs. It includes all interactions with strangers, friends, family members, neighbors, and the community at large. Our instilled behaviors, whether healthy or unhealthy, have evolved from a long personal story immersed in memories, feelings, losses, expectations, and perceptions of who, what, and how we should be in the world. This environment is the mirror that reflects our personal virtues and values, as shown in the diagram below.

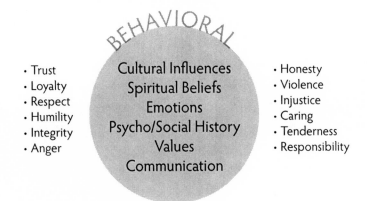

BEHAVIORAL

- Trust
- Loyalty
- Respect
- Humility
- Integrity
- Anger

Cultural Influences
Spiritual Beliefs
Emotions
Psycho/Social History
Values
Communication

- Honesty
- Violence
- Injustice
- Caring
- Tenderness
- Responsibility

THE CONSTRUCTED ENVIRONMENT

The constructed environment is what we create or alter as the product of our intellectual, economic, and social relationships to meet our physical, biological, and psycho/social needs. More simply, the constructed environment can be defined as how we construct our lives through the influence of our own nature, nurturing, and necessity.

Sorting out and prioritizing the "need to do" versus the "want to do" becomes increasingly complex in this environment. Sometimes, as the saying goes, we are our own worst enemies. In our determination to make adjustments, we may also find ourselves coming to the realization that less truly is more.

Our nature relates to the personal actions we construct that are linked to our beliefs. Have you perhaps said, "It is in my [their] nature to…?" Within the constructed environment dwell our unique idiosyncrasies, habits, routines, and ways of "doing" that influence and organize our day-to-day planning and decision-making.

Some individuals hold tightly to routines such as taking a morning run despite all kinds of weather or attending church or synagogue regularly. Tasks may also be organized by days of the week. So ingrained are these routines that nothing short of dying can alter them because it is in our nature to observe them. By example, I heard my husband once comment to a friend that I was generous "almost to a fault." That is my nature. It is also in my nature to keep learning.

Nurturing is a part of our constructed environment that involves routines, tasks, and commitments that also influence how we construct the priorities of our days. Attending children's sporting activities, recitals, plays, graduations, and reading bedtime stories are all nurturing validations.

Caring for family, friends, and volunteering our services in various ways is also a nurturing activity that must be configured into how we construct our days and hours, yet nurturing responsibilities and obligations that we "must" do take a toll on our well-being.

Necessity, taking on certain responsibilites because few, if any, options may exist, is perhaps the most challenging influence on the constructed environment for individuals and families. Almost inevitably, a cascading effect is put into motion. This first- or second-order change assaults our nature and nurturing while imploring action, often taking a tremendous toll on our wellness even in the short-term.

Perhaps work or home situations must dramatically change or a personal/family illness surfaces. These stressors complicate our ability to meet our commitments not only to ourselves but to others. The following Constructed Environment diagram summarizes these key points.

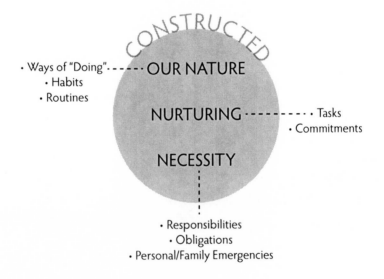

THE NATURAL ENVIRONMENT

Our natural environment includes time and all its dimensions as well as space and energy. These three elements influence us holistically, as they should. Both joys and sorrows are often integrally linked to each element separately and collectively.

Time can be described through calendar, clock, and historical contexts, each rife with emotional and even spiritual implications. Consider these common questions: "When is it the right time?" "Is the timing right?" "How timely is it?"

Recently, I followed a daily Doonsebury cartoon series in our local paper in which a young woman and her grandmother were stranded in a snowstorm along a highway. As the snow piled up over their car, the young woman began to think her life might end so she texted her boyfriend, asking him to marry her. From her perspective, it was definitely the *right time*, but you might say her *timing* was not the best, though it certainly was *timely*.

Contemplating the 1996 article by Dr. Avery I referred to earlier, I suggest that at the *time* his article was published, it did not ignite overwhelming action because other supposedly "salient" priorities were at the forefront of nursing education in the United States. Now, however, our world view has expanded exponentially, and the *timing* of this information is definitely salient and perhaps imperative. What's more, there should be no question that ecological wellness in nursing *isn't timely!*

Space is more than the spacial awareness we have with regard to our home or work locations. It is also about our personal space—how much or how little we have in the context of the natural environment. Where can we go to find ourselves? Is it through our own front doors and into our carefully constructed living spaces, or is it in the open places of nature? What about your space at work? Often it is communal or even non-existent.

Also, what defines too much space or not enough for your physical, emotional, and spiritual needs? Culturally, human beings are very particular about this. We prefer to maintain certain distances between ourselves and other people even as we talk, so much so that if someone stands too close, our personal space feels violated. Perhaps when visitors come to stay for an extended time, their influence shifts the dynamics of our personal space and the routines within it. Although we are often glad to see them arrive, we tend also to be thankful to reclaim and return our own space back to the norm when they depart. Also, have you known someone who may have been described as "emotionally distant" or perhaps "too close to the situation"? Space relates to an emotional dimension as well.

Energy is very influential across all environments. It relates to the energy we need to sustain our space as well to get to and from it, which may require transportation covering a number of miles. It is also relevant to our emotional and spiritual energy and our challenge to honor those dimensions as well. I ask again, where do you go to find yourself? Where do you go to replenish and renew these dimensions? What drains your energy? What/who are your resources to replenish this energy? In 1984, Bubolz and Whirin made the following timeless assumptions with regard to energy:

- Supplies of human energy, physical and psychic, are limited
- Any alteration in the flow of energy—matter, information, and other resources—requires adaptive change
- The behavior of an individual family member may require additional energy inputs and/or outputs by other family members as well as energy outputs for obtaining additional support and care for that individual
- High energy demands create "energy sinks" whereby adaptive creative behavior may not be

possible, resulting in still greater stress on the family (5)

Recall also the tremendous long-term energy depletion that occurs under the weight of a significant loss and subsequent movement along the grief journey. Recall how even one particularly challenging twelve-hour shift can affect the level of our energy in the subsequent days ahead. Forty-eight hours may not be sufficient restorative time before returning for another shift. Is it not surprising then that current nursing literature and workshops highlight "compassion fatigue"? This is an excellent example of identifying the pain but failing to look elsewhere for the problem. Compassion is nourished by an energetic soul. Compassion thirsts for this energy. Without replenishing ourselves from the well of soul, we have a severe case of compassion dehydration, which is far more serious than simply compassion fatigue.

The Natural Environment diagram below summarizes these key elements.

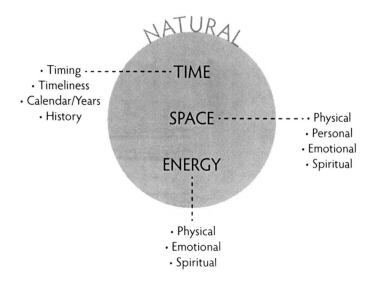

Conclusion

Let's revisit the word "courage" with the help of Mark Nepo, who reminds us that the word comes from the Latin *cor*, literally meaning "heart." The original use of the word "courage" means "to stand by one's core," a belief embraced in many traditions (*Finding Inner Courage,* 10). Living from our core or center is what enables us to face whatever life has to offer. Mark asks us to think about how we find the way to our core, stand by our core, and then sustain the practice of living from our core. This is to live courageously with our hearts wide open.

You will notice that the ecological wellness survey I include on the next page asks us to name what "encourages" our wellness in each environment. To "encourage" means to both inspire confidence and impart strength, to keep reaching for our best selves. So we must continue to do our "homework" because, as the saying goes, "Home is where the heart is."

The next chapter invites you to courageously explore the inter-relationships of the behavioral, constructed, and natural environments as they enjoin within the context of a sacred space. If we are true to our path of caring, this is where our healing presence is most at *home*, and so are we.

ECOLOGICAL WELLNESS SURVEY

This three-part reflective worksheet is intended to help you:

1. Identify what encourages as well as discourages your wellness in each environment
2. Identify any adaptation press you experience within the behavioral, constructed, or natural environments
3. Determine what environment you would like to identify to begin with, assuming you want to start making changes for your wellness

Part One: Beneath each environment listed below, please briefly note encouraging and/or discouraging wellness factors that affect you holistically.

Behavioral Environment
Encouraging:
Discouraging:

Constructed Environment
Encouraging:
Discouraging:

Natural Environment
Encouraging:
Discouraging:

(CONTINUED)

Ecological Wellness Survey

(cont. from page 53)

Part Two: Please explore the following questions below.

1. Adaptation press can be defined as environmental demands that are exerted upon a system that may encourage and/or *force* adaptation regardless of an otherwise steady state. Within the three environments, can you identify any "press" to change?

2. Are one or more environments affected?

Part Three: Please explore the following questions below.

1. In what environment (if any) would you like to see a wellness change begin?

2. A wellness change I would like to address is...

References

Avery, A. 1996. "Eco-Wellness Nursing: Getting Serious about Innovation and Change." *Nursing Inquiry* 3: 67–73.

Bubolz, M., J. Eicher, and S. Sontag. Spring, 1979. "The Human Ecosystem: A Model." *Journal of Home Economics* 71(1): 28–31.

Bubolz, M., and A. Whirin. Jan., 1984. "The Family of the Handicapped: An Ecological Model for Policy and Practice." *Family Relations* 33(1): 5–12.

Carper, B. 1978. "Fundamental Patterns of Knowing in Nursing—Practice Oriented Theory—Part 1 Nursing. *Advances in Nursing Science* 1(1): 13–23.

Nepo, M. 2007. *Finding Inner Courage.* San Francisco: Conari Press.

Olson, S. 1988. "Hospice Adminstration: A Lifecycle Model." *American Journal of Hospice and Palliative Medicine Care* 5(40): 41–47.

Ramen, R. N., M.D. 2000. *My Grandfather's Blessings—Stories of Strength, Refuge, and Belonging.* New York: Riverhead Books.

Watzlawick, P., C. E. Weakland, and R. Fisch. 1974. *Change— Principles of Problem Formation and Problem Resolution.* New York: W. W. Norton.

Suggested Readings

Leininger, M., and J. Watson. 1990. *The Caring Imperative in Education.* New York: National League for Nursing.

"Do unto others as you would have them do unto you." Luke 6:13. It is both simple and possible. — Maggie, R.N., 32 years

This quote is from Pierre de Chardin: "Someday, after mastering the winds, the waves, the tides and gravity, we shall harness for God the energies of love, and then for a second time in the history of the world, man will have discovered fire." — Marion, R.N., M.S.N., AHN-BC, 29 years

This quote is from Dorothy Allison: "Behind the story I tell is the one I don't. Behind the story you hear is the one I wish I could make you hear." — Jane, R.N., 28 years

This quote is from Phillip Moffitt: "It is a beautiful and mysterious power that one human being can have on another through the mere act of caring. A great truth, the act of caring is the first step in the power to heal." — Laurie, R.N., O.C.N., 27 years

Believe in the incredible strength inside yourself and care for each individual as if they are family. — Shauna, nursing student

I have kept this quote by Rainer Marie Rilke on my calender for the last twenty years. It has kept my heart focused on what I believe about nurses and nursing. Although I am retired now, the poem still keeps my heart on "loving the question": "Have patience with everything unresolved in your heart and try to love the questions themselves...Live the questions now. Perhaps then, someday far in the future, you will gradually, without even noticing it, live your way into the answer." — Sister Jean, R.N., 55 years; also submitted by Mary, R.N., 44 years

4

DWELLING IN THE CENTER—
ENTERING THE SPIRITUAL SPACE

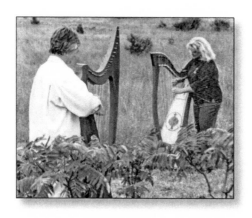

*The friend who can be silent with us in a moment of
despair or confusion, who can stay with us in an hour
of grief and bereavement, who can tolerate not-knowing,
not-curing, not-healing and face with us the reality of our
powerlessness...makes it clear that whatever happens in
the external world, being present to each other is what
really matters.*

HENRI J. M. NOUWEN, *THE THREE MOVEMENTS*
OF THE SPIRITUAL LIFE

I will open the door of this chapter with a question, and I will close it with a comment. It is my hope that whatever you find meaningful in between will guide reflection and resonate with your own unique wellness journey.

It is here that I ask men and women in the nursing profession to enter the deeper water—not to drown, but rather to float and reflect on what cost there is to nursing if we submerge our own humanity. This deeper water is also intended to validate the wisdom of our collective compassion. It takes courage to extend our reach into the space where answers are first heard with the heart.

The question I want to open with is this: *How well are you on the inside of yourself today?* More than ten years ago, Dr. Blair Justice, a professor of psychology at the University of Texas-Houston School of Public Health, called for a major reformation in our perception of health as "the absence of disease," suggesting rather that the sense of an individual's well-being is the "best measure" of individual health. In his article "Being Well Inside the Self: A Different Measure of Health," he noted that

> Most intriguingly, a number of people are reporting on adult health surveys that they are well although they, in fact, have disease, disability, or some other kind of disorder. They do not deny that something is wrong with their bodies, but they do perceive themselves as possessing a sense of health and being well inside themselves at a deeper layer than physical (61).

This same article referenced numerous large longitudinal multi-country studies analyzing mortality data demonstrating that "self evaluations of our health predict mortality above and beyond…the presence of health problems, physical disability, and biological or lifestyle risk factors" (63).

Another focus of wellness derives from hospice and palliative care. Balfour Mount, a prominent Canadian surgical oncologist and academic who is considered the "father" of palliative care in North America, began asking his patients, "When were you last well?" The answers he received repeatedly demonstrated that terminal patients could die "well" when they held on to a core sense of nonphysical health even when the body experienced terminal illness and pain (Cohen and Mount 40.) The hospice movement from its inception has indeed offered a holistic wellness focus as an exemplar for the broader health care arena (Olson, *Your Gift*, 7).

So, I ask again: How well do you feel on the inside of yourself today, on a scale of 0-5, with 0 being *not well at all* and 5 being *very well*? This simple question in and of itself shifts the perspective from *illness* to *wellness*. The diagram below represents the interrelationship of the three environments that overlap and interact continually. Perceiving yourself as "very well" or "not well" has everything to do with the synergistic nature of the behavioral, constructed, and natural environments in *balance* at the center. Their total effect is greater than the sum of their individual influences. As you truly listen to the answer your heart proclaims as to how well you do or do not feel, know that you have already entered the "deeper water."

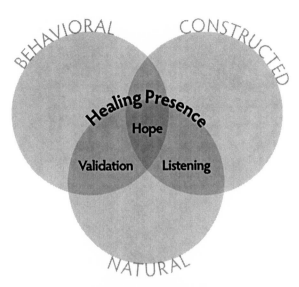

SPIRITUAL SPACE
Includes an awareness of soul, higher being, presence of something/someone greater, synergism, grace, emergence of best self, and peace.

ENTERING THE SPIRITUAL SPACE

The fundamental meaning of the word "spirit" derives from the Greek word *pneuma* meaning "air" and the Latin *spiritus* meaning "breath." It is interesting that these are the two most basic needs we have for survival. I imagine that our spiritual space is akin to the home of the soul where all the windows are wide open so that we can inhale peace and exhale the stillness we need to reclaim our life's path. Let me clarify that I am not referring specifically to a religious context here. The silent harmony between our souls and our lives is bidding us to the sacred work of nursing, one soul to another.

Henri Nouwen in *Reaching Out* eloquently describes the essence of this "soul to soul" harmony: "When we think about the people who have given us hope and have increased the strength of our soul, we might discover that they were not the advice givers, warners, or moralists, but the few who were able to articulate in words and actions the human condition in which we participate and who encouraged us to face the realities of life" (60–61).

In "The Art of Caring for the Spirit," the authors inform us that like all aspects of our being, our spirituality is dynamic and always changing, because "Just as there is an ebb and flow to life, there's an ebb and flow to our spirituality as well. It is natural for us to experience varying levels of spiritual comfort and distress along the continuum of our spiritual journey. Ironically, times of spiritual distress can be opportunities for profound spiritual growth" (Holland, Hagstrom, and Ziegenhagen 30).

The times when we stumble and lose our emotional/spiritual footing are when one or more of our environments may be rife with demands and challenges that feel overwhelming. Yet there are those who courageously step into the fray as a healing presence, helping us regain our footing and balance. How is this possible? These caring friends, family members, or sometimes even strangers are most at home in their own spiritual space and have the capacity to attune—come into harmony—with both the person and the situation. They intuitively validate our best selves by listening and holding our hope until we can hold it once again for ourselves.

Within this spiritual space, there might also be an awareness of a higher being or the presence of something/someone greater than we might comprehend in the moment. Ultimately, this is also the home of our own healing presence revealed through our astute ability to listen behind words, to validate both moments and journeys, and to hold another's hope.

Presence

Some time ago, I discovered the following story as part of a collection of "This I Believe" essays aired on National Public Radio. "The Power of Presence" by Debbie Hall, a psychologist in San Diego's Naval Medical Center Pediatrics Department, related her experience of being "hurled" into an ambivalent presence when a friend's mother unexpectedly died. Part of her wanted to rush to her friend's side, but another part of her didn't want to intrude. An insightful friend advised her to "Just go. Just be there." Debbie did, and she never regretted it. Since that formative moment, she has not hesitated to be in the presence of others for whom she could "do" nothing. Debbie offered this perspective:

> Presence is a noun, not a verb; it is a state of being, not doing. States of being are not highly valued in a culture which places a high priority on doing. Yet true presence or "being with" another person carries with it a silent power—to bear witness to a passage, to help carry an emotional burden or to begin a healing process. In it there is an intimate connection with another that is perhaps too seldom felt in a society that strives for ever-faster connectivity—the healing power of connection created by being fully there in quiet understanding of another conveys that none of us are truly alone. The power of presence is not a one-way street—not only something we give to others. It always changes me, and always for the better.

When we first meet someone new, a sense of their presence is quickly discerned. Our perception of their presence may also change over time as we have more interaction with them. For me, there have certainly been brief times when my presence wordlessly conveyed anger, love, happiness ambivalence, fear, sadness, and even anxiety. But generally, with time, there is a constancy in the manner and stride of a person's presence that we come to know, anticipate, cherish, or maybe even dread.

For instance, you really become aware of the dignity and light of human presence when you are in the company of a charismatic person. This presence inspires you with an awareness of the natural balance this individual holds between their personality and their vision. These individuals carry a huge spirit that deeply illuminates their nature to reach out and encourage us. They reflect a lovely harmony and resonance of their true self both inside and out, offering a light of inspiration and vision for what is possible.

In March of 2012, I attended the 11th Annual Advanced Practice Nursing Conference in Lansing, Michigan. Geradine Simkins, R.N., M.S.N., a certified nurse midwife, gave the closing keynote address reviewing her many years of activism for the care of pregnant women and infants in underserved countries and in the education of nurse midwives. Her presentation theme was "Activist and Change Agent: The Right Person, In the Right Place, at the Right Time."

Geradine's global journey as an activist was a universal message of compassion, courage, and commitment inspiring the hundreds of nurses who attended her session. Our collective gratitude resulted in a standing ovation that reminded me of Ralph Waldo Emerson's quote that "Our chief want is someone who will inspire us to be what we know we could be."

Geraldine's gift to the audience that day inspired us to "see" how the vision of just one person can bring about change if we tenaciously stay true to our path.

Healing Presence

Deep speaks to deep, spirit speaks to spirit and heart speaks to heart.
Henri J. M. Nouwen, *Finding My Way Home*

The concept of "presence" within the context of nursing was first introduced in 1976 and described as "a mode of being available or open in a situation with the wholeness of one's unique individual being; a gift of self which can only be given freely, invoked or evoked" (Paterson and Zderad 122).

Through subsequent years, the growth of the holistic nursing movement has both promoted and advocated for a more comprehensive platform of nursing interventions that strengthen what is essential in a nurse's caring role. In 1994, the *Journal of Holistic Nursing* published an excellent article titled "The Healing Process of Presence" written by two nurses, Maggie McKivergin and Jean Daubenmire. Together, they strongly advocated for the necessity of healing healthcare systems that begin "understanding the principles behind healing ourselves and others in ways that offer integration and balance in the dance of compassionate human interaction" (66).

McKivergin and Daubenmire were motivated to action by a keen awareness of major problems occurring at two levels. First, that patients were experiencing fragmented and impersonal care in a current disease care system, and second, that this same disease care system was dramatically in need of being healed itself.

In response, these authors stressed the urgency of reclaiming the concept of "presence" as the essence of nursing practice that readily blended into nursing theories of care, nurse/patient relationships, energy systems, self-care, and health as expanding consciousness (65). A problem surfaced, however, in the variable terms and definitions they presented, confounding the simplicity of the very word "presence."

They identified "true presence," "presence in the moment," "unconditional presence," "psychological presence," and "therapeutic presence." They also identified "physical presence," defined as "being there," in contrast with "psychological presence," which was defined as "being with."

These authors chose "therapeutic presence" to reflect interpersonal relationship skills at the physical and psychological levels in their two-day course entitled "The Essence of Therapeutic Presence" in which caregivers explored dimensions of self and learned ways to enhance the nursing experience by bringing more energy, insight, and meaning into their own lives as well as those of their patients (69–71). Outcomes of over 150 caregivers who participated in the course included a deeper appreciation of the whole of the patient's experience as well as of personal and intrapersonal dynamics of presence with self, patients, and other nurses (78).

Finally, the significant theoretical constructs of Jean Watson's Caritas Consciousness as part of the fourth Caritas Process I introduced in Chapter One resonate most intimately with both the spiritual space and healing presence. She embraces the use of a "phenomenal field" as holding the subjective and intersubjective meanings of both participants as an "authentic spirit to spirit connection that radiates *beyond* the moment for both the nurse and the patient" (Watson 79). Her remarkable influence in teaching and scholarship has called many nurses back to embrace the heart of what they came to nursing for in the first place.

Within the ecological model of wellness, I prefer to use the term "healing presence" to represent the core of our best selves within a spiritual space. I believe there is great beauty quietly carried in the arms of healing presence as the life force of nursing. This healing presence cannot be faked or acquired like an accent. It comes from within us as strength and grace, gently illuminating a deeper meaning to our lives and the lives we touch.

From my viewpoint, healing presence encourages movement beyond an already saturated, albeit necessary, therapeutic- and skill-oriented focus in both nursing and medical education. For a moment, stop reading and simply ask yourself, "Do I want to be *therapeutic* or *healing* with myself?" Feel the difference?

In March of 2012, I presented my ecological model focusing on spiritual space and healing presence at a Michigan statewide nurse practitioner conference. I asked for the attendee's thoughts, questions, and/or comments regarding the difference between *therapeutic* and *healing* presence. Two attendees articulated the consensus of the larger group, offering these thoughts:

- ◆ "Therapeutic presence is unidirectional. Healing presence denotes an exchange *between* individuals." (Laura, Kalamazoo, MI)
- ◆ "Healing presence involves more compassion and strength giving as opposed to therapeutic presence, which ensures that treatment is provided competently and appropriately." (Linda, Grass Lake, MI)

Simply, if we perceive every encounter with our patients as an opportunity to heal and to extend love, we are in alignment with the dignity and grace of our soul's calling and our profession. That's all. And ultimately, that's everything.

In *The Gift of Healing Presence,* Jim Miller defines healing presence as "A deeply conscious and compassionate sharing of moments with another person that naturally encourages movement toward greater wholeness" (8). Healing derives from the root word *haelan,* which is the origin of our word "whole." Miller reminds us that we don't *do* healing presence. We are to *be* healing presence guided by several key assumptions:

- Healing presence requires consciousness. It doesn't just happen—we intentionally make it happen.
- Our healing presence is compassionate.
- Healing presence is quietly confident that whatever the life situation of the other person, there is potential for wholeness.
- Our state of being exists nowhere other than in the present moment completely concentrated on the well-being of the one in our care (9).

Our first step is to look not at the other person but at ourselves and to listen within. What influences within our own life stories helped form who we are today? What are our fears, joys, passions? Who/what inspires us? What have been our most profound experiences of caregiving and care receiving? Are we caring well for ourselves?

Inasmuch as healing presence is more art than science, Jim Miller and Susan Cutshall in *The Art of Being a Healing Presence* offer seven suggestions for bringing healing presence into the spiritual space while acknowledging that we each will have our own unique ways of doing this:

1. *Open yourself.* Begin not with the other person but with yourself. Become present to your uniqueness, humanness, prejudices, brokenness, and wholeness. Own your life story.

2. *Intend to be a healing presence.* Intend to promote healing in its many forms.

3. *Prepare a space for healing presence to take place.* Clear a space to interact with calmness and privacy. Prepare a space within by clearing yourself of your personal expectations of what the other should be or do.

4. *Honor the one in your care.* Approach those in the spiritual space with dignity and worth. Respect their natural and unique healing capacity by honoring their individuality, equality, humaness, separateness, and sacredness.

5. *Offer what you have to give.* Freely and simply make available what you have to offer, realizing it's up to the other or others to accept it or not. Offer hope with your firm belief in them and your willingness to follow their lead.

6. *Receive the gifts that come.* Accept with a grateful heart what is yours to receive. This may include living your life more fully, uncovering your genuine self, receiving your own healing, finding personal satisfaction, and/or realizing you have made a difference.

7. *Live a life of wholeness and balance.* There is more to life than being a healing presence, so live your days fully, caring for your own needs, setting appropriate boundaries, encouraging your own growth, and nurturing a loving attitude

toward life, including the sacred dimension. Affirm and live your truth, being grateful for possibilities now and for those that are still waiting for you (74–75).

The Triad of Healing Presence: Listening, Validation, and Hope

Three key aspects are inherent in healing presence. Listening and validation are related to communication, and hope is closely aligned to commitment. All three are integrally linked and must be held as precious keys to unlocking the door to healing—ours and others'.

Listening

In 1998, I wrote about four realms of listening used when offering bedside musical care that included the patient, the environment, their own inner self, and the spiritual space ("Bedside Musical Care," 572). I often tell my students that their harp "always knows" what is going on inside them. Thus, if they are not centered on the "inside," how can they help someone with their music on the "outside"?

Henri Nouwen reminds us that "Listening is not a technique but rather an art. It must be developed and requires our full and real presence. When we listen through and through, it makes the individuals familiar with the terrain they are traveling through and helps them go the way they want to go" (*Reaching Out*, 95).

An example of listening "through and through" is conveyed by a nurse in the following home visit:

I have gathered my supplies and stand at the door to leave when Sarah realizes this is her "last chance" to say something she had not wanted to mention in the course of the last hour we have been together caring for her husband. Now she stands next to me saying that "Something has been weighing heavy" on her mind. I listen to more than her words as tears well up in her eyes. She holds clasped hands close to her chest as she begins to talk about being alone "after he..." but she cannot bring herself to finish the word that we both know is inevitable. I listen. I will not and cannot leave in this moment. For a while longer, we stand together—more than just physically—in her grief. Sarah continues to talk. I listen deeply with all that I am. Then, after a few moments of silence, she sighs and gently says, "Thank you. This helped a lot!" We share a heartfelt hug as I leave. Again, I am in awe, witnessing the strength of the human spirit in moments like this.

I suggest that this example reflects that listening involves more than our ears. With intention, we hear things also with our eyes and our hearts.

VALIDATION

I purposely introduced validation earlier in Chapter Two because it is essential in all aspects of our communication. Now, however, it is integral to both listening and hope as part of the healing triad. The above example gently reflects the nature and nurturing power of validation. There are times when very few words are spoken yet *everything* is understood. Staying alert with eyes, ears, and heart in these moments reveals opportunities to companion another human being in their unfolding journey. In the context of Sarah's story above, let's review again the attributes of true validations.

1. *Putting aside judgment.* This requires letting go of judging the delays in the leavetaking and choosing not to judge Sarah's timing in bringing up her feelings. The nurse's flexibility requires "bending" time to make it work for healing.

2. *Committing to Sarah's best self.* Sarah's capacity to rise to the occasion when obstacles seemed impossible was validated through the nurse listening and trusting that Sarah was able to find her own best words to convey her grief without any interruptions or advice giving.

3. *Appreciating both the moment and the journey.* The emotional fullness within those few minutes for both the nurse and Sarah reflected the importance of appreciating the moment in which Sarah found the courage to speak of her burdens and the pain of her journey as it was at that moment.

4. *Witnessing both the moment and the journey.* "Being there" and being fully present wordlessly validated Sarah's grace, courage, and fears of both the moment and the grief of her days to follow.

5. *Being honest and gentle.* Honest and gentle encouragement called for a "heartfelt hug" as part of the leavetaking. The nurse's gentle attentiveness was an honest reflection of the respect she had for Sarah and all that weighed heavily in the moment.

However brief, this was also a sacred space in which both the nurse and Sarah felt something greater guiding the moment.

If you have not experienced such a moment, I hope you will at some point in your professional journey. It will be forever remembered, because it reflects why you are a nurse. It is a validation that caring is the most essential and most universal essence within ourselves and others.

Hope

"La esperanza muere última."

Recall that hope relates to commitment. You and I have hope when what we desire is accompanied by a commitment to the expectation of fulfilling that which we desire. Milton Mayeroff also reminds us hope is not to be confused with wishful thinking and unfounded expectations or passive waiting for something to happen from the outside. Rather, it is an expression of a present alive with possibilities, energy, and action.

When we make a commitment to "hold hope" for ones we care about and care for, it extends from the now into the future with the sure belief that an individual's deep resilience will guide them to what is yet possible. In *On Caring*, Mayeroff says, "It is not simply hope for the other, it is hope for the realization of the other *through* my caring: and therefore an important aspect of hope is courage. Such courage is found in standing by the other in trying circumstances" (25–26).

In their book *Finding Hope*, Ronna Jevne and Jim Miller tell us that hope is amazing! We can't touch it, but we can definitely feel it. We can't physically see it by itself, but we can hold it and carry it for ourselves and others. Hope doesn't weigh anything, but it can ground and anchor us.

Hope is also paradoxical. We can live under extremely adverse conditions and have a great deal of hope, yet those who may seem to have everything going right in their lives may feel little or no hope. We can even be dying and have much that we're hopeful about.

There is no substitute for hope. While closeness and love may encourage it, they will not duplicate it. By contrast, two basic situations contribute to feelings of hopelessness—uncertainty and captivity. When we are uncertain, we fear that things will change in some way we don't want them to. When we feel captive, we dwell on the impossibility of things changing. In both cases, we seem to be confronted with losing control of the future and of the hope that sustains us (Jevne and Miller 6–10).

Also, when we tie hope to something that really matters to us, we have more energy and endurance to move forward. This connection gives our days meaning in a very personal way. In our search for what is meaningful in life, right next to it we find what gives us hope (Jevne and Miller 53).

Three brief examples support this definition of hope. First, a scholarly thesis in 1998 by Kathryn Gray informed advanced practice nurses about the multidimensionality of hope as it applied to the elderly, validating that hope is indeed a vitally important health care parameter that could serve as a basis for establishing quality of life dimensions. Additionally, she noted that in the primary care setting there are opportunities to instill, maintain, and restore hope as part of a nurse's clinical practice (7).

Second, Dr. Jan Romand's doctoral research with bereaved parents after the accidental deaths of their teenage children found what she refers to as "posttraumatic" hope. This was a conscious choice to go on with their lives, facilitated by allowing interventions with others and by initiating interventions themselves. She also found that other bereaved parents provided validation, guidance, and hope, serving as role models for a positive future (243).

Finally, the translation of the Spanish at the beginning of this section is "Hope dies last." This was the title of an article written by Alex Kotlowitz about his ninety-six-year-old dear friend Studs Terkel, whom he interviewed shortly before his death. Terkel, the well-known author of *Hard Times: An Oral History of the Great Depression*, commented, "So here we are at a crossroads. In a strange way, I'm hopeful. Without hope, you can't make it. And so long as we have that hope we'll be okay. Once you become active helping others, you feel alive...You become a different person. And others are changed too" (51).

CONCLUSION

It will be interesting to follow the current unfolding drama within healthcare reform. Trends to establish patient "medical homes" and the electronic medical record are purported to decrease costs while improving continuity of care, data consolidation, and access. Yet who will track the essential issue of decreased or minimalist caring that is likely to be buried under these other priorities?

The future of nursing education must have a unifying narrative in helping students guide and honor their own wellness "upstream" pre-clinically. A holistic understanding of how they maintain their well-being from an ecological perpective both honors and guides their own potential to be a healing presence first for themselves and only subsequently for their patients. Suffice it to say that a balm for healing is best used sooner rather than later.

An article I wrote in 1984 entitled "Hospice Care: A New Option for Nursing" suggested that nurses need an acute power of observation, an exquisite sensitivity to patients' needs, and an infinite capacity for compassion (51). Today, at both our professional and personal levels, we are increasingly confronted with ever more demanding personal life challenges, changes, and losses while also caring for others.

Now, in 2012, I would revise my original quote of over a quarter century ago to convey that what nurses need today is an acute power of self-observation regarding their own wellness, an exquisite sensitivity to their own needs and self-care, and an infinite capacity for *self*-compassion if they are to do more than survive this profession and instead thrive.

At the beginning of this chapter, I promised to begin with a question and end with a comment. The comment is this: *Be encouraged!*

Webster's College Dictionary defines "encourage" as inspiring with courage and hope. We know people whose presence in and of itself feels encouraging even when no words are spoken. John O'Donohue suggests that one of the most beautiful gifts in the world is the gift of encouragement. When someone encourages us, they help us over a threshold we might never have crossed on our own. When times of great uncertainty seem overwhelming and friends come with words of encouragement, they bring light and lightness that helps us find the stairs and the door out of the dark. It is not simply their words or gestures that help but rather their whole presence—their healing presence—enfolding us and helping us find the concealed door (*Eternal Echoes*, 62).

Encouragement also helps us to engage and trust our own possibilities and potential. O'Donohue also reminds us that sometimes we are unable to see the special gift of encouragement that we bring to the world, yet some of our deepest longings are exactly the voice of our gift calling us to embrace hope with courage and humility. This voice alone knows where our path leads. To follow the path that encourages us holds fulfillment, while failing to do so unwittingly sows seeds of regret (63).

Offering an excerpt from his poem "For a Nurse" published in *To Bless the Space between Us* (142) seems very applicable to this moment.

> *May you never doubt the gifts you bring;*
> *Rather, learn from these frontiers*
> *Wisdom from your own heart.*
> *May you come to inherit*
> *The blessings of your kindness*
> *And never be without care and love*
> *When winter enters your own life.*

Finally, *may you be encouraged* to dwell in the spiritual space of your own life. As you become a healing presence for yourself, so shall you be for others.

References

Cohen, S. R., and B. M. Mount. 1992. "Quality of Life in Terminal Illnes: Defining and Measuring Subjective Well-Being in the Dying." *Journal of Palliative Care* 8: 40–45.

Gray, K. 1998. *Hope and the Elderly Individual: Clinical Assessment and Hope-Fostering Strategies for the Advanced Practice Nurse in Primary Care.* Unpublished scholarly thesis. Michigan State University.

Hall, D. Dec. 26, 2005. "I Believe in the Power of Presence." *All Things Considered.* NPR. http://www.npr.org/templates/story/story.php?storyId=5064534.

Holland, E., A. Hagstrom, and M. B. Ziegenhagen. 2012. "The Art of Caring for the Spirit." In *Your Gift: An Educational, Spiritual, and Personal Resource for Hospice Volunteers.* Sharon Olson, ed. Traverse City, MI: Seasons Press.

Jevne, R., and J. E. Miller. 1999. *Finding Hope.* Fort Wayne, IN: Willowgreen Publishing.

Justice, B. 1998. "Being Well Inside the Self: A Different Measure of Health." *Advances in Mind-Body Medicine* 14: 43–73.

Kotlowitz, A. Jan., 2009. "Studs Terkel: Hope Dies Last." *AARP—The Magazine* 52(1).

Mayeroff, M. 1971. *On Caring.* New York: Harper Row.

McKivergin, M. J., and M. J. Daubenmire. 1994. "The Healing Process of Presence." *Journal of Holistic Nursing* 12: 65–81. Online at http://jhn.sagepub.com/content/12/1/65.

Miller, J. 2010. *The Gift of Healing Presence.* Ft. Wayne, IN: Willowgreen Publications.

Miller, J., and S. Cutshall. 2001. *The Art of Being a Healing Presence.* Fort Wayne, IN: Willowgreen Publications.

Nouwen, H. 1975. *Reaching Out—The Three Movements of the Spiritual Life.* New York: Doubleday.

O'Donohue, J. 2002. *Eternal Echoes—Celtic Reflections on Our Yearning to Belong.* New York: First Cliff Street Books/ Harper Perennial edition.

O'Donohue, J. 2008. *To Bless the Space between Us: A Book of Blessings.* New York: Doubleday.

Olson, S. Dec., 1984. "Hospice Care: A New Option for Nursing." *The Journal of Practical Nursing* XXXIV(2): 50–52.

Olson, S. 1998. "Bedside Musical Care: Applications in Pregnancy, Childbirth and Neonatal Care." *Journal of Gynecologic and Neonatal Nursing* 27: 569–575.

Olson, S. 2012. "The Ecology of Wellness; Hospice As an Exemplar." In *Your Gift: An Educational, Spiritual, and Personal Resource for Hospice Volunteers.* Sharon Olson, ed. Traverse City, MI: Seasons Press.

Paterson, J. G., and L. T. Zderad. 1976. *Humanistic Nursing.* New York: John Wiley & Sons.*

Romand, J. 2010. *Postraumatic Hope: The Lived Experience of Bereaved Parents 4–10 Years after the Accidental Death of Their Teenage Child.* Unpublished dissertation, Union Institute and University.

Watson, J. 2008. *Nursing—The Philosophy and Science of Caring.* Revised edition. Boulder: University Press of Colorado.

Webster's College Dictionary. 1995. Costello, R., ed. New York: Random House.

*Continuing their efforts on behalf of nurses world-wide, the authors now offer their book complete in eText form as a free download at http:// www.gutenberg.org/files/25020/25020-8.txt.

Suggested Readings

Miller, J. 2003. *The Art of Listening in a Healing Way*. Ft. Wayne, IN: Willowgreen Publications.

Nepo, M. 2007. *Finding Inner Courage*. San Francisco, CA: Conari Press.

This quote comes from Helen Keller: *"Many persons have the wrong idea about what constitutes true happiness. It is not attained through self-gratification but through fidelity to a worthy cause."* — Penny, R.N., 13 years

This quote comes from Clara Barton: *"I have an almost complete disregard of precedent, and a faith in the possibility of something better. It irritates me to be told how things have always been done. I go for anything new that might improve the past."* — Mary, R.N., B.S.N., 47 years

This quote comes from Daniel Pesut, Ph.D., R.N.: *"Are you content to be pushed by the past or do you prefer to be pulled by the future?"* — Marylee, M.S.N., R.N., N.P., 40 years

This quote by Robert Kennedy, based on a line from George Bernard Shaw's play *Back to Methuselah*, is my favorite. It told me not to accept things the way they are, whether it is one patient's situation or the health care system in general: *"There are those who look at things the way they are and ask why? I dream of things that never were and ask why not?"* — Margaret, R.N., 42 years

This quote comes from Clara Barton: *"An institution or reform movement that is not selfish must originate in the recognition of some evil that is adding to the sum of human suffering, or diminishing the sum of happiness."* — Barbara, R.N., retired

5

REFORMATION
AND RENAISSANCE

*I've learned that loving yourself requires a courage un-
like any other. It requires us to believe in and stay loyal
to something no one else can see that keeps us in the
world—our own self-worth.*

MARK NEPO, *THE BOOK OF AWAKENING*

Much has changed for nurses both educationally and
within the work environment. This chapter focuses on the
deeper context of our profession's reformation. The treatise has
been nailed to the door for everyone to read, and each of us
will initially experience these changes positively or negatively,
with neutrality a non-sequitur.

Facing these changes will require perseverance because
this significant moment holds something much greater than
reform. A renaissance is also underway. It is slowly gaining the
brilliance of a sunrise on our professional horizon, carrying
the hope we need for a new day as nurses.

Webster's College Dictionary defines *renaissance* as "A movement or period of vigorous artistic and intellectual activity—a re-birth—a revival." We nurses have a rich opportunity to midwife these changes. However, it will not be an easy delivery. In many of us, the unconscious soul of our nursing practice must first be resuscitated.

Dr. Fred Otte, professor of vocational and career development at Georgia State University in Atlanta, suggests that soul, spirituality, and vocation can't be separated, relating that, "When people are out of touch with the deepest parts of themselves, they and their employers lose a vital resource" (Henry and Henry 68).

When caring stops, does staffing really matter? This is the question Kathy Douglas, founder and president of the Institute for Staffing Excellence and Innovation, poses in sharing the widening concern that caring is compromised in healthcare today. "When it comes right down to it," she says, "no matter how modern, sophisticated or efficient staffing programs are, if the individuals who are executing the care are not qualified, engaged, and able to offer the caring necessary for healing, the whole system can unravel quickly. At its very essence staffing works because of the people who are staffed" (415).

She continues, "Intuitively we know it is not a good thing when someone who is delivering care is out of balance, emotionally spent, or has lost their capacity for compassion. But how often does it change our staffing or assignments and do we take actions to help the individual get back in balance?" (415).

THE REFORMATION BEGINS

In early 1984, renowned nurse scholar, researcher, and educator Dr. Patricia Benner wrote, "If we are to humanize care in the midst of highly technical medicine, we must master the technology. We must also critique the technology and not view it as the ultimate resource in recovery, dignity and health. As an antidote to the purely technical view of health and power, we must understand and unleash the power of caring, the power of excellence" (*From Novice to Expert*, 220).

Fast forward to 2010. Dr. Benner's scholarship was again instrumental in directing a long overdue study of the current status of nursing education. This was at the request of the Carnegie Foundation for the Advancement of Teaching, which had funded a previous study of nursing's educational endeavors forty years earlier.

"The profession of nursing in the United States is at a significant moment" is the very first sentence of the introduction in *Educating Nurses—A Call for Radical Transformation* by Benner, Molly Sutphen, Victoria Leonard, and Lisa Day (1). This groundbreaking book is the culmination of the Carnegie research study, which informs us that the demographics of major impending nursing shortages combined with overwhelming challenges within nursing education are calling into question the health and well-being of our own profession.

The research accurately illuminates the ever-burgeoning information of nursing science, bioethics, physiology, and other classroom subjects as well as multifaceted and demanding clinical responsibilities. This situation is further complicated by the shortage of both nurses and nursing faculty. To meet these challenges, the authors assert that schools, service providers, and the profession itself must change. They suggest faculty and students make four shifts in their thinking and approach to nursing education. I follow each recommendation with an ecological wellness model interpretation in italics.

Shift one: from a focus on decontextualized knowledge to an emphasis on teaching for a sense of salience, situated cognition, and action in particular situations.

Context should refer to the "wholeness" and influence of all environments. Salience is meaning, yours and theirs, that yields to the ebb and flow of deeper understanding and the actions that follow.

Shift two: from a sharp separation of clinical and classroom teaching to integration of classroom and clinical teaching.

Utilizing an ecological foundation of understanding for students' personal lives, their ways of being, and the choices they make within each environment offers early integration for a deeper and more diverse understanding of caring in the clinical setting.

Shift three: from an emphasis on critical thinking to an emphasis on clinical reasoning and multiple ways of thinking including critical thinking.

The ecological model widens the lens of understanding the reasons for patterns and actions taken in each of the interrelated environments.

Shift four: from an emphasis on socialization and role taking to an emphasis on formation (Benner et al. 89).

The spiritual space we enter for ourselves and with patients is where healing presence is formed and nurtured. It is the door to transformation for both the giver and the receiver of caring as they become partners in the dance of true reciprocity.

This ecological wellness model for nursing education has not been specifically named as such until now, yet I believe it will be a positive influence guiding us along the path of a most remarkable reniassance in our own lives and our profession.

Reniassance—A Clarion Call

I am drawn to the emphasis on both the use of formation and transformation the four authors use in *Educating Nurses*. Formation speaks to the "now," fostering the unfolding process of a deeper understanding that transforms our future ways of thinking, being, and doing.

Transformations of mind, body, and spirit reveal a new, deep, and "lived vision" we have for ourselves. They speak both to the now and the future and a new "lived truth." Recall the use of the word "transformation" in John Schneider's grief model reviewed in Chapter Two. He reminds us that life itself is a transformative experience and a form of freedom, helping us to regain a spiritual openness in the empowering of our *best self* (304).

Transformation of knowledge that is then seen as truth is articulated through the wisdom of Parker Palmer, who in 1993 presented the Michael Keenan Memorial Lecture at Berea College, Kentucky, entitling his address "The Violence of Our Knowledge: Toward a Spirituality of Higher Education."

He asked us to consider that every way of knowing becomes a way of living and suggested that a spirituality of learning or a *"transformed understanding of knowing"* derives from the following four components:

- *Learning is personal.* In contrast to modern objectivism, the wisdom of spiritual traditions tells us that truth is personal. It drives our understanding of knowing to a deeper level and we embody it both through "walking our talk" and "talking our walk."
- *Learning is communal.* Here, movement toward truth is a cooperative endeavor involving

conflicts that we must reach consensus on, yet we must also break that consensus when some new observation has been made or a more powerful interpretation has been offered.

- *Learning is reciprocal.* We are not only seeking truth; truth also seeks us. At the heart of all great knowing is a sense that learning encompasses a personal quality eager to connect the knower with the knowing.

- *Learning is transformational.* Truth changes us, and there is no way to evade it. Knowing, teaching, and learning will transform individuals if that same knowing, teaching, and learning are guided by the images and norms that the knower has been trying to articulate (1–2). To state this more simply, there is a silent harmony between the inside and the outside of our "being," and it is this harmony that transforms us.

THE ROLE OF GRATITUDE

It is impossible to hold resentment and gratitude in your hand at the same time.

S. OLSON

How can we begin to introduce these aspects of knowing into undergraduate nursing programs as a foundation from which we plant the seeds not just for care but for caring? I suggest that often we misplace the "ing" in our philosophical dimension of contemporary nursing practice which represents our *inner gratitude* for the privilege of sharing in the most personal moments of illness, suffering, pain, joy, and sorrow of another human being. How often at the end of our workday do we take a few moments to thank our assigned patients for the privilege of caring for them? How often do we neglect to thank our colleagues for the "extra hands" they gave us during our shift? Remember that gratitude is also another form of validating an individual's worth.

Did you know that even "gratitude" is now being researched? Drs. Blair and Rita Justice at the University of Texas Health Center at Houston report that gratitude is good for you, *really* good for you.

In their article "Giving Thanks—The Effects of Joy and Gratitude on the Human Body," they report that researchers have found that when we think about someone or something we truly appreciate and experience the feeling that goes with the thought, the parasympathetic calming branch of the autonomic nervous system is triggered. This pattern, when repeated, bestows a protective effect on the heart. Also, the electromagnetic heart patterns of volunteers become more coherent and ordered when feelings of appreciation are activated. The authors also note that bringing attention to what we appreciate in our lives causes more positive emotions to emerge, which leads to beneficial alterations in heart rate variability. Perhaps it isn't surprising, then, that individuals who keep gratitude lists are more likely to make progress toward important personal goals (1).

The authors relate that gratitude can also be a total body experience and beyond, meaning the deepest and widest gratitude comes from the soul and that part of the brain, the amygdala, that registers "soul" experiences. By example, they offer this description:

"So when we look at snow-capped peaks or golden swatches of changing aspen or the Milky Way at night from high in the Rockies, our souls sing and our bodies are suffused with streams of dopamine and serotonin, the gifts of gratitude" (2).

CARING AS SOUL WORK

Sooner or later, something calls us to a particular career path. Does your work represent a job to you, or a vocation for you? At a very young age, I knew I wanted to be a nurse. Later, I understood it was my calling, my vocation, an expression of my values and beliefs about what it is to be a human being in this world.

By contrast, "a job" implies work of necessity, "a must do," often primarily to meet financial obligations. In this circumstance, a person may or may not be invested in giving "their best," particularly if the job itself is unsatisfying. Such work may also be soul diminishing (Henry and Henry 69.) Yet at times the terms may be variable, as when people honestly say, "I love my job!"

The following story conveys just how vital our attitude toward our work is.

> *Three prisoners worked every day at hard labor in a rock quarry breaking up large stones. Each was asked what motivated them to work under such harsh conditions. The first replied that it was to pay for his wrongdoing and that soon he would be released. The second replied that if he broke up so many pounds of rock, he would be paid a small amount of money each day. The third replied that the stones he was breaking were going to be used to make a beautiful cathedral in their town someday.*

Linda Gambee Henry and James Douglas Henry in *Reclaiming the Soul in Health Care* offer insight to the prisoner example from both the old and new paradigms in the way we approach work:

- The old paradigm derives from seventeenth century perceptions of an objectified and quantified universe in which work was viewed as boring and machinelike with pay as the driving incentive.
- By contrast, the new paradigm reflects the belief that the universe is an interrelated system intricately ordered and purposeful. If we believe and participate in work that is an evolving and creative process, each job, no matter how small, holds meaning and contributes to the whole (41–42).

The authors define soul as a "mysterious, living, organic energy serving as a unifying, holistic web of connectedness throughout the universe that is touched by *experience*." They offer the following five questions to help us discern when we are doing soulful work (70). I hope you will take some time to reflect on your own answers.

1. What are you doing when time seems to fly?
2. What activity captivates your childlike playful passion?
3. What type of work summons your energy and enthusiasm?
4. What undertaking becomes the focus of your creative impulse?
5. What essential gift(s) do you wish to give to the world?

I would add one last question:

6. When was the last time you were engaged in this type of activity?

Your answer to this question will be an insightful reflection of how well you honor your own self-care.

Using the metaphor of a spider web, Henry and Henry convey how the sum total dynamic energy of the entire web is greater than the individual strands. For example, when a team of people, an organization, or a social unit connect to souls, the result is a synergism, as in (1+1=3). Also, when we pull on one of the web's strands of the universal soul, whether for better or worse, we affect everything else because everything interrelates (14–15). The authors suggest four specific ways to enhance soul in healthcare. Again, I will relate an ecological wellness perspective in italics following each point.

First, we enhance soul in healthcare by promoting individual depth, meaning, value, and growth. Organizations encouraging individual expression and creativity enhance the soul and are more productive.

Deepening personal meaning, value, and fostering growth must be integral to the educational process pre-clinically. There is the fertile soil where we develop personal appreciation and respect for the diversity of life influences, challenges, change, loss, and transformations within each of the environments. This is the prescient "terra firma" for clinical rotation because students have applied the ecological wellness model to themselves through listening, holding hope, and validating their own unique path of growth holistically as well as that of their fellow students.

Second, we enhance soul in healthcare by advancing career satisfaction. Soul thrives on job satisfaction and the work of our passion.

How satisfied we are at work in large measure reflects the influence of what we do outside the workplace to renew and replenish ourselves. The most effective programs in self-care <u>simplify</u> people's lives. The importance of space as discussed within the natural *environment is essential. To give oneself some "space" or separateness for transitions from work to home as well as space to engage in activities that are restorative is literally soul food.*

Third, we enhance soul in healthcare by honoring diversity in both thought and experience. The soul flourishes where diversity is honored outwardly and inwardly.

Understanding the whole context of any life experience immerses us fully in an ecological perspective whether we intend it or not. Soul reaches beyond gender, skin color, or socio-economic status to feel the true pulse of our humanity.

Fourth, we enhance soul in healthcare by valuing and nurturing community. Synergism occurs when there is a deep connection with others (16–17).

Without a contact point in the form of a person or community, a spark is just that. It will go nowhere. It will kindle nothing. The spiritual space is both the spark and the kindling as one. It is interaction with self and others. It is also reciprocal because as we give, we will also receive, whether it is realized at the moment or at some later time. It is where truth finds us.

Such concepts represent a huge stride forward on the road to renaissance. If hospitals are beginning to embrace this philosophy, nursing education surely would do well to join them in partnership while preparing students to become employees in a "soul-full" environment.

Conclusion

One last metaphor on soul, which I use with students in relation to their willingness to enter the spiritual space where the soul of healing presence is most at home. I often ask students to consider a matchstick as representing themselves and to hold it in one hand, while holding the matchbox, representing their soul, in the other. The lesson is clear: both the matchstick and the matchbox must be present in order for a spark to occur.

You see, if we have lost touch with our souls, there will be no spark, no matter how we may delude ourselves. We need our souls in order to create the spark to illumine healing. It is not a coincidence that Florence Nightengale first carried a lamp. The textbooks came later.

In *The Book of Awakening*, Mark Nepo tells an interesting tale about chickens and their need for light. Simply, if chickens don't get enough light, they start pecking at each other. Before farmers realized it was a lack of light that prompted the pecking, they thought pecking was simply the nature of chickens. Mark explains:

> The truth is that humans are no different. The removal of light causes us to peck at ourselves and each other. Once the pecking begins, we are called to three forms of work: stop the pecking, heal the wounds, and seek out more light. The eternal squabble has always been which of these efforts comes first: governance, medical and social healing, or education.

> Ironically, the more removed we are from light, the less faith we have in its restorative powers. All our energy is spent strategizing how to peck or how to avoid being pecked. The first task of any newcomer, regardless of their community, is to learn the pecking order.

Mark's profound final point is that it's not the free range of our thinking and the depth of our feelings that are dangerous but rather the fact that our minds and hearts are often incubated in the dark. The conclusion: we just need to hold each other more fully in the light (141).

Mary Raymer and Gary Gardia, authors of *Leadership in Everyday Life*, encourage each of us to be that light of leadership in our own lives. This means "leading with our values, finding the courage to act, and using personal insight to identify our strengths and challenges, in essence leading our whole selves to wellness" (x).

Ultimately, it could be said that this quest is about finding our soul's voice and thus reclaiming the truth that has been seeking us all along.

References

Benner, P. 1984. *From Novice to Expert—Excellence and Power in Clinical Nursing Practice.* Menlo Park, CA: Addison-Wesley Publishing Co.

Benner, P., M. Sutphen, V. Leonard, and L. Day. 2010. *Educating Nurses—A Call for Radical Transformation.* San Francisco: Jossey-Bass.

Douglas, K. 2010. "When Caring Stops, Staffing Doesn't Really Matter." *Nursing Economic$* 28(6): 415–419.

Henry, L. G., and J. D. Henry. 1999. *Reclaiming the Soul in Health Care.* Chicago, IL: American Hospital Association Press.

Justice, B., and R. Justice. 2003. "Giving Thanks—The Effects of Joy and Gratitude on the Human Body." *HealthLeader.* www.uthealthleader.org/archive/mind_body_soul/2003/givingthanks-1124.html.

Nepo, M. 2000. *The Book of Awakening—Having the Life You Want by Being Present to the Life You Have.* San Francisco, CA: Conari Press.

Palmer, Parker J. 1993. "The Violence of Our Knowledge: Toward a Spirituality of Higher Education." The Michael Keenan Seventh Memorial Lecture, Berea College, Kentucky. http://www.kairos2.com/palmer_1999.htm.

Raymer, M., and G. Gardia. 2011. *Leadership in Everyday Life—It Really Is All About You.* www.leadershipineverydaylife.com.

Schneider, J. M. 2012. *Finding My Way—From Trauma to Transformation: The Journey through Loss and Grief.* Traverse City, MI: Seasons Press.

Webster's College Dictionary. 1995. Costello, R., ed. New York: Random House.

I've worked in cardiac stepdown, recovery room, and helped in all nursing departments, ER, and ICU as well. To all the new nurses that I come to know, I give them my own saying on a jewelry box trinket. It is "Compassion is the key." Never lose the compassion you will give and possess to assist others in their sickness/hospitalization. — Melissa, R.N., B.S.N., 12 years

My nursing practice has been inspired by "But for the Grace of God there go I." I always reflected on how I would handle this situation if I were the patient or the patient's family member. I have always put the patient first in all of my decisions. I have been blessed to have chosen a career that I have personally received much more in return than I have given." — Maxine, R.N., 39 years

This quote is from an unknown author: "Compassion fatigue: when you have built your identity on carrying the burdens that rightfully belong to others." — Catherine, Psy.D., APRN-BC, 45 years

This quote is from Florence Nightingale: "Nursing is an art: and if it is to made an art, it requires an exclusive devotion as hard a preparation as any painter's or sculptor's work; for what is having to do with a dead canvas or dead marble, compared with having to do with the living body, the temple of God's spirit? It is one of the Fine Arts: I had almost said, the finest of Fine Arts." — Muriel, R.N., parish nurse, 50 years

6

The Future of Nursing: Three Transformative Paths of Compassion

A vision without a task might be a mirage; a task without a vision can be a drudgery, but a vision with a task brings hope to the world.

Inscription on a church wall

The word that defines our profession, "nurse," derives from the Latin and means "to nourish," which in turn means "to promote growth." There is such eloquence in the simplicity of this word. It distills both our personal and professional essence into two questions regarding the path we walk in the labyrinth of our lives. First, does this profession nourish you? And second, does it promote your growth?

In the previous chapter, I indicated that reforms are happening within our profession. Indeed, seeds have already been planted for the renaissance. I speak of this nursing renaissance as offering new professional directions, new paradigms of caring, and new educational advancement options. The door of many possibilities is opening for both today's and tomorrow's nurses.

Dr. Tommie Nelms at Georgia State University contributed these words in 1990 that are even more relevant today:

> Ultimately within these reconceived notions of curriculum that espouse freedom, choice, existence, and transcendence in nursing education, there is no curriculum until each individual reflects and creates personal meaning of the planned learnings. A curriculum only becomes a curriculum as it is experienced by the individual creating meaning and releasing potential (285).

Dr. Margaret Newman, a nurse theorist pioneer in her vision of health as expanding consciousness, notes that many theorists are now echoing the call for integration of all types of knowledge for nurses in the educational process (*Health As Expanding Consciousness* website). She stresses, however, that integration is a step in the overall cyclic scheme of things but that it is not enough. We must move to a realm of nursing that includes and transcends all the realms that have gone before. This is a shift to a more inclusive level of wholeness whereby transformation comes about by attending to *pattern*. She says

> We cannot understand the unity of nursing knowledge just by integration of the parts because each part contains the whole; each part is reflective of the whole. Mind and matter are not separate, interactive parts; they are different dimensions of the whole and unbroken movement of reality. What is needed is transformation to another realm; a shift to a more inclusive level of wholeness. Transformation comes about by attending to pattern. It is integral to nursing. It is based

on relationships, it includes the focus (i.e., the client) [and] the environment, and its meaning permits a jump from what is seen and heard to the larger context and from the explicit to the implicit ("The Pattern That Connects," 5–6).

I believe Dr. Newman is trying to help us understand that all movement in our personal and professional realms relates to patterns, and that once they are comprehended as a whole, they can become our guides to healing action. As she suggests, this unitary approach to caring is an authentic, interactive, and receptive relationship that centers on meanings of life patterns within the wholeness of a person's life. Nurses practicing within this perspective have found that their own lives are enhanced and transformed by the experience as well.

Once again, I draw from another important osteopathic assessment premise as it pertains to patterns. It is, "Do not mistake motion for action." The dictionary, of course, defines motion as *movement*. However, action is "the accomplishment of a thing usually over time."

When patients present with pain, their assessment includes observing motion in all types of activity (i.e., walking, standing, sitting, bending) as well as prone and supine positions. Both structural asymmetry and compensatory motion may be evident. Therefore, my treatment priorities for restricted *motion* are to restore balanced musculoskeletal *action* and resolve the pain.

Unfortunately, the longer dysfunctional motion patterns exist, the more challenging it is to meet such goals. Isn't that true elsewhere in our lives as well? When the compensatory motion patterns we develop don't seem to work anymore, we feel out of balance and perhaps even experience physical, emotional, and spiritual pain. Indeed, this is "going through the motions" of living. Only reconnecting with what is meaningful and relevant holistically will render the call to action that we desperately seek ("The Pattern That Connects," 1).

This chapter highlights three remarkable transformative paths gaining momentum with patterns that both "walk the talk and talk the walk" of our nursing profession. They are nurse coaching, gender neutral nursing, and faith community nursing. Their compassionate patterns call us to be more inclusive in our ways of knowing how to foster healing action. As Rumi poignantly observed, "Each forest branch moves differently in the breeze, but as they sway they connect at the roots."

TRANSFORMATIVE PATH NUMBER ONE: NURSE COACHING

Coaching is not a new concept to our profession. Patricia Benner, in fact, identified the second of her seven domains of nursing practice as the "teaching-coaching function." In her book *From Novice to Expert—Excellence and Power in Clinical Nursing Practice*, she stressed, "We will be over-simplifying this role if we look only for information giving or formal 'precepts' because the more significant learning lies in coping with illness and mobilizing for recovery, which includes ways of being, ways of coping, and even new possibilities" (78–79).

There is a swell of interest in nurse coaching that is beginning to crest, thanks particularly to help from holistic practice nurses. What started in 2000 with Wellcoaches™ Corporation, a strategic partner of the American College of Sports Medicine, is now the gold standard in coaching competencies in healthcare, fitness, and wellness industries. As of 2010, this corporation had the largest community of coaches in healthcare worldwide, training more than one thousand coaches per year (Moore and Tschannen-Moran xiii).

Thus it is very timely to begin infusing nursing education coaching curricula with a two-fold purpose. First, for nurses' own improved concept of wellness, and second, for the positive impact this will have in both role modeling for and educating their patients.

In 2002, nurse authors Susan Schenk and Kay Hartley proposed a new role for nurses in an article titled "Nurse Coach: Healthcare Resource for This Millennium." They defined the nurse coach role as "an expanded professional interaction based on mutual respect of the knowledge and skills that both nurse and client bring to the situation" and noted that "the concepts of self-efficacy, stages of change, and motivational enhancement are integrated in the coaching or partnering role" (15).

The authors stressed the importance of client-focused as opposed to illness-focused interactions, with nurse coaches considering each individual's medical, emotional, and social concerns that translate into a plan for behavior change that honors the complexity of each individual. They stressed that nurses are uniquely qualified to provide a structure and approach to custom-fit wellness goals for each client (19).

Another influential article by Susan Luck, "Changing the Health of Our Nation—The Role of Nurse Coaches," stressed that this is indeed an important time for the nursing profession to expand its visibility. She said, "As health and wellness coaches, nurses are the trusted professionals emerging as pioneers on the vast frontier of our nation's health care reform. Nurses possess the essential tools to create health coaching programs that embrace our nation's renewed focus on wellness and patient-centered care" (78).

In looking to the future, Susan believes that coaching presents nurses with creative opportunities to be leaders in transforming health care. She states, "Perhaps more empowering is the knowledge that health and wellness education may be the greatest gift to the future generations and nursing's most enduring legacy" (80).

Why such interest in coaching? In large measure it has to do with *Wellness Initiative for the Nation*, a document crafted by the Samueli Institute in 2009 in collaboration with leaders in the fields of health policy, health promotion, and integrative health care practices with the goal of moving America toward a greatly expanded wellness and prevention infrastructure. This initiative generated increased interest in wellness coaching by many professional groups that is ongoing today.

Holistic Nurse Coach Leadership. Both interest and concern have grown considerably regarding coaching standards specific to nursing practice. Nurse coaching builds upon a holistic nursing foundation already focusing on relationship-centered care that enhances the healing process (Luck, Dossey, and Schaub 9).

In 2010, the American Holistic Nurses Association (AHNA) took a leadership role in establishing the AHNA Nurse Coach Task Force to address professional nurse coaching and to explore a national holistic nurse coach certification process. This organization subsequently drafted the "White Paper: Holistic Nurse Coaching" and presented it at the National Professional Coaching summit sponsored by Harvard University to demonstrate and educate other disciplines about how holistic nurses, with their scope of practice and strongly defined professional ethics, were in a position to lead this national effort for the emerging coaching model (Hess, Bark, and Southard 9).

Other coaching education efforts are ongoing. For example, Sigma Theta Tau International and the International Council of

Nursing offer six free continuing education credits including a workbook entitled "Coaching in Nursing—An Introduction" by Gail Donner and Mary M. Wheeler.

Nurse Coach Insights. Dr. Barbara Dossey, author, Nightingale scholar, and well-established holistic nurse coach, notes, "Our life's challenge is to understand how to handle the double-edged sword of capacity—our ability to give and contribute to society and also to find ways to care for and coach ourselves so we do not burn out. When we understand this, we can be a coach for clients at a deeper level" (Luck 79).

Dr. Darlene Hess, a holistic nurse coach and nurse educator, anticipates a next step to include coaching skills in educational programs for nurses. She relates, "I foresee coaching skills being added as an essential requirement for nurses to have. When that occurs, nursing programs across the country will be adding coaching skill training to their curricula" (Luck 79–80).

Nurse practitioner Dr. Eileen O'Grady shares this awareness: "I knew that people did not need more information about wellness as much as support in living the lives they truly want to be living. Wellness coaching helps people make sure what they value most is regularly expressed in their lives" (Hanson 9).

Nurse Coaches within the Ecological Wellness Environments. As you will see below, the 2012 scope and standards of care for holistic nursing practice gleaned from the American Holistic Nurses Association Position Statements harmonize beautifully with the ecological wellness environments presented in Chapter Three:

BEHAVIORAL

♦ They value the whole person

- They enjoy mutual respect with their patients and one another
- They facilitate healing
- They alleviate suffering
- They take responsibility for nurturing each other

CONSTRUCTED

- They create environments that foster optimum mind/body/spirit healing
- They offer and take advantage of scholarship opportunities that assist in understanding and evaluating the holistic nature of the human experiences of health, healing, illness, and recovery
- They contribute to society at large through initiating and supporting actions to meet the social and health needs of the public

NATURAL

- They consider the health of the ecosystem in relation to health, safety, and peace

SPIRITUAL SPACE

- They embrace a professional ethic to holding hope for growth and healing for self and others through a variety of techniques designed to enhance the mind's capacity to affect bodily functions and symptoms (1–4)

The culminating chapter of *Educating Nurses—A Call for Radical Transformation* by Patricia Benner and colleagues summarizes twenty-six recommendations with the intention to encourage a transformation of nursing education to meet today's needs. Recommendation number eighteen is "Support faculty in learning how to coach." The authors acknowledge that coaching is routinely part of teaching in the clinical setting yet add that it should be extended to the classroom, which would strengthen problem-solving in situations that more closely resemble what future nurses will encounter with patients (Benner et al. 225).

TRANSFORMATION PATH NUMBER TWO: GENDER NEUTRAL NURSING

There is a need for many hands and this may be nursing's shining moment.
DR. CATHERINE GILLISS, PRESIDENT,
AMERICAN ACADEMY OF NURSING

The positive influence men bring to the nursing profession is still being submerged in a quagmire of stereotypes, misperceptions, and organizational adjustment disorders. However, I am optimistic their important contributions will be validated in the renaissance of our nursing future. Much is already changing for the better.

Recently, I reviewed the findings of a 2004 online survey titled "Men in Nursing" by Hodes Research representing 93% RNs and 7% nursing students. On average, the RNs surveyed had been in the profession for 14 years with 16% reporting 20 to 25 years (12). Nearly 45% of those surveyed planned to return to school for an advanced degree as part of their long-term career goals (17). The survey summary provided these key conclusions:

- Men choose nursing for much the same reasons as their female counterparts, primarily to help others and for growth opportunities the profession offers. Many spoke of nursing as a "calling," not just a profession, and offered numerous comments about being able "to make a difference."

- Key challenges to men in the nursing profession include stereotypes and cultural adaptations required for entry into a traditionally female profession. Misperceptions include that the profession is "not appropriate" for men, that they must not have been able to make it into med school, or they must be gay.

- Many respondents disliked the use of "male nurse" and felt it contributed to the problem.

- Most of the men surveyed were not actively involved in initiatives to attract more men to nursing careers.

- Four-fifths of the men surveyed said they would do it all over again (38–39).

It is also important to validate the compelling insights men shared in the remaining ninety-seven pages of the document. I found these verbatims to be more insightful than the actual number-crunching section. Indeed, vicariously, the various ecological environments and the spiritual space were woven into their lived experiences.

Gender Neutral Nursing within the Ecological Wellness Environments. In the voices that follow, we hear the understory of their lives as nurses:

- "Many families don't consider a nursing role for their sons."

- "...I have learned there are three types of nurses: RN's, LPNs, and male nurses. I am an RN, not a male nurse."

- "By understanding the group of men whose readiness to change, not only their own career, but what they value in life, we can identify a large and eligible group of men, unchallenged by the existing institutional structure."

- "We are fathers, husbands and sons, community volunteers, and leaders. We teach, we volunteer our time as scout leaders, baseball coaches, and community activists. We like to hunt, fish, and watch baseball, but most importantly, we can lend a hand to people who need us in their most difficult time."

- "Forget the archaic gender stereotypes. It's okay to be nurturing/compassionate and be a man."

- "It's not just a job. It's a proud and noble commitment to life and humanity."

- "I wish this had been an option I'd considered earlier in life" ("Men in Nursing," 47–135).

CONSTRUCTED

- "Many textbooks refer to 'she' as the nurse and lack pictures of men in nursing."

- "Our hospital celebrated National Nurses Week by giving each nurse a lovely flower, a nice heart-shaped note pad, and a free facial! This organization has an unusually large number of men in nursing and still fails to recognize the insult that those gifts represent."

- ◆ "Hollywood still does a pretty lousy job in how males in the nursing profession are portrayed in movies and on television."

- ◆ "Although there have been men in nursing for a very long time, I feel like a pioneer cutting-edge career frontiersman."

- ◆ "Do not become a male nurse. Just become a nurse and make an impact on nursing."

- ◆ "I'm basically proud to be a nurse, but I am tentative in expressing it because it forces one to wade through the stereotypes" ("Men in Nursing," 43–125).

Natural

- ◆ "Twelve-hour shifts on consecutive days are murder at any age. Documentation takes a tremendous amount of time and takes away from patient care."

- ◆ "I don't have enough time in the day to finish all my work" ("Men in Nursing," 120 and 123)

Spiritual Space

- ◆ "You can have compassion and empathy and make a difference in someone's life. These qualities are human, not gender."

- ◆ "It's not as hard as you think, and it is the best feeling when you know you have really done something that helps another person."

- ◆ "Nursing has made me a better husband, son, and member of my community. In nursing I've worked with dysfunctional and functional families, and in each case, I'm able to learn something valuable. There has never been a day in my twenty-five-year career that I have regretted being a nurse."

+ "It has helped me to become a whole person. I've been able to work at the bedside, in the ICU, in hospice and now in informatics—all within the same profession. Few other professions allow such flexibility when it comes to career changes."

+ "The experiences with the variety of people I have worked with, learned from, taught, and taken care of are memories for life. Nursing has given me the opportunity to help better people's lives and a better understanding of my inner self. I have found inner peace within myself through being a nurse."

+ "I get what others search endlessly for—personal validation and human affirmation" ("Men in Nursing," 67–134).

Do many of these quotes seem gender neutral? Perhaps that is exactly my point. What binds us through compassionate understanding is always stronger than the tension that divides.

In 2011, an article by the Robert Wood Johnson Foundation (RWJF) entitled "Human Capital: Male Nurses Break through Barriers to Diversify Profession" highlighted the overlooked role of men in the history of the nursing profession. Men attended the world's first nursing school in India in 250 B.C. and were instrumental in helping to start a hospital for providing care during the Black Plague epidemic (1).

In another publication by RWJF titled "How to Dramatically Increase the Formal Education of America's Nursing Workforce by 2020," the lead sentence on enhancing diversity reveals that nursing education has a poor record of recruiting and retaining male students in part because schools lack faculty and staff role models and mentors. As of September, 2011, the RWJF reported that men comprised just over seven percent of all RNs (6).

Men's Nursing Leadership. The American Assembly for Men in Nursing (AAMN) was established in 1974 with a mission of providing a framework for nurses as a group to meet, discuss, and influence factors that affect men as nurses. The organization's objectives are these:

- To encourage men of all ages to become nurses and join together with all nurses in strengthening and humanizing health care
- To support men who are nurses to grow professionally and demonstrate to each other and to society that increasing contributions are being made by men within the nursing profession
- To advocate for continued research, education, and dissemination of information about men's health issues, men in nursing, and nursing knowledge at the local and national levels
- To support members' full participation in the nursing profession and its organizations while using the Assembly for the limited objectives as stated above (1)

This organization continues strengthening connections for men choosing the nursing profession with its three-pronged approach of recruitment, retention, and concomitant promotion of men's health.

Academic Insights. As the recipient of the 2010 Best School for Men in Nursing Award from the AAMN, Duke University's School of Nursing reports that men comprise eighteen percent of its faculty and staff. These individuals believe the key to their success is a welcoming environment and team spirit. Assistant Professor John Brion, Ph.D., R.N., notes, "Men entering an overwhelmingly female environment develop 'role strain.' They don't know how to act, and they don't feel they belong. Having numerous male faculty and staff eliminates this strain" (RWJF, *Charting Nursing's Future,* 6). Additionally, this nursing school's outreach speaks directly to men through its campus chapter of AAMN.

TRANSFORMATIVE PATH NUMBER THREE: FAITH COMMUNITY NURSING

The spiritual life is about becoming more at home in your own skin.

PARKER PALMER, IN *THE BOOK OF AWAKENING* BY MARK NEPO

As you read about faith community nursing, I ask that you contemplate two questions. First, how would you define spirituality? Second, how does spirituality relate or not relate to your nursing practice?

In her book *Caring from the Heart—The Convergence of Caring and Spirituality,* Simone Roach reminds us that for all people of whatever faith persuasion, spirituality is an integral, holistic, dynamic force in human life for the individual and for the community. She suggests that spirituality has also become a kind of universal code word for the search for meaning and that this search is more than for individual identity; it is rather a search for the meaning of our personhood, our interconnectedness with others beyond our individual, biophysical experience. Simone maintains that we each have an awareness of this call within ourselves (11–12).

Another scholar, Paulette Burns, defines spirituality as "The process of striving for and/or being infused with the reality of the interconnectedness among the self, other human beings, and the Infinite, that occurs during a depth experience" (149).

Paulette's choice of the word "infinite" closely relates to the synergistic dimension of the spiritual space in which healing presence is most at home. It includes an awareness of soul, a higher being, a presence of something/someone greater than oneself, grace and serenity, and both emergence and validation of the best self.

Paulette also uses the words "depth experience" drawn from frequent references by the participants in her study who described a vividly specific moment in time in which they knew without a doubt that something profound had happened (145).

Elizabeth Mazzella, R.N., submitted her story for this book that poignantly reflects the wordless power of spiritual space:

I was a nursing student in clinical rotation in 2002, and while doing my clinicals, I had an experience that affected me deeply. I was assigned by my instructor to care for an elderly aphasic stroke patient, and I didn't think I was doing anything significant. All I had done was help her out of bed to a chair and provide basic care such as bathing. However, when it was time to leave and I went to say goodbye, she grabbed my hand and touched it to her cheek. Even though she could not speak, the look in her eyes said it all about how much I really had done for her. That experience gave me the motivation to make it through nursing school, and many

other like experiences I have had since have motivated me to
further myself in this caring profession so that I can play a
more direct role in the lives of my elderly patients. This hap-
pened to me ten years ago now, and I have never forgotten it.
I sometimes think about how we forget so many things that
happen to us in our lives, but remember others so clearly.

The second example happened to me many years ago and
affirms that such validations are indeed always remembered:

At our local hospital, I was providing bedside musical care
with my harp in a volunteer capacity for a woman who was
quite ill. I normally sit beside the bed to play, but due to many
pieces of equipment, I sat with my harp at the foot of her bed.
She was awake and appeared to be comfortable as I began
to play. Soon she closed her eyes and within a few minutes
extended a slow widening reach upward with both her arms
as if to embrace someone or something. She held them there
for perhaps thirty seconds, then gently lowered her arms to
her side. I continued playing for a few minutes longer, then
sat quietly. Soon she opened her eyes and looked at me, both
of us deeply understanding that no words had been neces-
sary. Everything had been heard and seen, and we were both
changed.

"Re-membering" can be thought of as experiencing a significant moment that re-connects us to the core of our best self.
Simone Roach believes that core, the center of our spirituality,
lies within the heart. As the primary organ of our being, it is
the center of life, the determining principle of all activities and
aspirations; it embraces everything that comprises what we
call a "person." She says the heart is the ground of the soul,
the core or apex of our being (13).

Another voice, Parker Palmer, suggests that the aim of all spiritual paths, no matter what their origin or the rigors of their practice, is to help us live more fully in the lives we are given. In this way, whatever comes from a moment's grace that joins us to our lives and to each other is spiritual (Nepo, *The Book of Awakening*, 119).

Faith community nursing fully embraces this spiritual context as the heart of nursing in many communities both locally and globally. Yet care today is often provided through volunteer efforts, and advocacy for salaried positions commensurate with this nursing role is slow to develop. This in part is perhaps due to initial expectations that "a giving spirit should be its own reward."

Faith Community Leadership. The Rev. Dr. Granger Westberg, recognized as the founder of parish nursing, remains a respected pioneer in both holistic healthcare and identifying the interrelationships of religion and medicine. He held joint professorships in religion at the University of Chicago as well as in preventative medicine at the University of Illinois College of Medicine and is well known for two books still in print, *The Parish Nurse* and *Good Grief.*

During the 1960s and '70s, Dr. Westberg began establishing holistic care clinics in churches staffed by a physician, nurse, social worker, and pastoral counselor. These clinics set the stage for parish nursing to evolve in the 1980s. By 1986, he also saw the need for special training programs through the Lutheran General Hospital system in conjunction with developing congregational partnerships. Thus was born the Parish Nurse Resource Center, now referred to as the International Parish Nurse Resource Center (IPNRC). Located in Memphis, Tennessee, its mission is to equip parish nurses to serve as health catalysts in faith communities through ministries of wholeness and healing (1).

Another excellent resource is the Health Ministries Association (HMA), which has as its goal to encourage, support, and empower leaders in the integration of faith and health in local communities.

There are many wonderful resources now available for faith communities, yet the overarching guidelines of practice for nurses in these settings derive from the Amercian Nurses Association (ANA).

In January of 2012, the ANA and the Health Ministries Association co-published the second edition of *Faith Community Nursing: Scope and Standards of Practice*. This document defines faith community nursing as "a practice specialty that focuses on the intentional care of the spirit, promotion of an integrative model of health and prevention and minimization of illness within the faith community." Further, "Such practitioners consider the spiritual, physical, psychological and social aspects of an individual to create a sense of harmony with self, others, the environment and a higher power" (1).

This new edition reviews sixteen standards that reflect the specialty's professional values, priorities, practice directions, and a framework for practice evaluation, with each standard measured by specific competencies that serve as evidence-based compliance.

Faith Nursing Insights. As mentioned earlier, I presented "The Ecology of Wellness for Nurses" model in draft form in 2012 at the Michigan Council of Nurse Practitioners Annual Conference in Lansing, Michigan. During my session, I invited the attendees to write down their thoughts or questions on this model as well as any quotes they might like to contribute for the book you are holding now.

Laura, a nurse practitioner, wrote:

Entering the spiritual space is what strengthens my core. Achieving that spiritual depth and breadth has taken years of daily devotional time. Yet I find that I lose the sense of my own spiritual health when I lose sight of God's vision of me—his beloved child.

Another attendee, Pat, wrote:

I have been a parish nurse since the summer of 2001, but it seems like just last year. It is an immensely rewarding and fulfilling ministry. The challenge involves trying to help people understand what we do. My credentials are R.N., M.S.N., P.N. (Parish Nurse), and it is this last one that renews me.

More recently, Vicki contributed a quote that is particularly relevant:

I felt the call to go into nursing in 1967 prior to graduating from high school. After receiving my LPN, I went to Newport Hospital School of Nursing, graduating in 1979 with a diploma in 1982 as valedictorian of the class. I say that humbly because I was in all remedial programs in high school and never thought I was capable of being a nurse. When I say that God directed my path, He opened doors for me then and continues to bless, protect, and lead me in my career...I have been nursing forty-five years and still love my profession...

The Faith Community Nurse within the Ecological Wellness Environments. Within the ecological wellness model, nurses incorporating faith community scope and standards of practice do the following:

BEHAVIORAL

◆ Integrate ethical provisions into practice
◆ Collaborate with patients, spiritual leaders, members of the faith community, and others
◆ Coordinate care delivery
◆ Interact with and contribute to the professional development of peers and colleagues

CONSTRUCTED

◆ Provide leadership
◆ Consider safety, effectiveness, cost, and impact on practice, planning, and delivery of services
◆ Integrate research into practice
◆ Implement the specified plan, evaluate their own nursing practice in relation to professional practice standards, and evaluate progress toward attainment of outcomes
◆ Attain knowledge and competency that reflect current nursing practices
◆ Systematically enhance the quality and effectiveness of faith-based community nursing practices
◆ Use prescriptive authority in accordance with state and federal laws and regulations where applicable

NATURAL

◆ Seek space for office location and services
◆ Assess time commitments as well as volunteer versus paid staff positions

- Determine energy needs to recruit volunteers and to assess program development and implementation requirements

SPIRITUAL SPACE

- Promote holistic healing with intentional care of the spirit
- Seek to create a sense of harmony with self, others, the environment, and a higher power

Faith community programs contribute significantly to many communities within different religious denominations and settings, yet "faith" is the gossamer thread connecting them to the greater good of humanity regardless of race or creed. As I reflect on the word "faith" in the larger context, I ask, is it not possible that the wholeness of this profession is held by "Faith" with a capital "F"?

It is Faith in caring and compassion; Faith in the humanity we bring to the bedside; Faith in the healing side of life while treating illness; and most profoundly, Faith as the complete trust that we, each in our own way, live the Word and Hebrews 3–13.

CONCLUSION

Together, the three transformative paths of nurse coaching, gender neutral nursing, and faith community nursing continue to both widen and lengthen the direction of our nursing profession. Each ultimately will hold personal lessons in humility.

Mark Nepo in *Finding Inner Courage* validates this humility when he refers to the "curious journey through the sweet labyrinth we call being alive":

You see, somewhere along the way, I realized that all the separate conversations are part of one conversation, and all the different questions are part of one inquiry, and all the colorful beings who ask, suffer, talk, and listen are part of one common element of being that binds us to the human family. And that element is precious and resilient. It can save our lives. I now accept that only by staying in this conversation together can we find the love and truth that helps us live. Without each other, we miss much of what we know. Without the courage to face each other and hold each other, we remain broken and adrift. It seems simple, but staying in conversation in this way is the source of joy. Our job is to nourish the spark of life we each carry inside (276).

Please consider that our lives may not revolve around great moments but rather great moments revolve around us as we courageously extend our reach for hope on behalf of another human being.

REFERENCES

American Assembly for Men in Nursing. http://aamn.org/aamn.shtml.

American Holistic Nurses Association (AAMN) Position Statements. 2012. 1–4. http://www.ahna.org/resources/publications/positionstatement/tabid/1926/default.aspx.

American Nurses Association and Health Ministries Association. Jan., 2012. *Faith Community Nursing: Scope & Standards of Practice.* Second edition. www.nursingworld.org.

Benner, P. 1984. *From Novice to Expert—Excellence and Power in Clinical Nursing Practice.* Menlo Park. Addison-Wesley Publishing Co.

Benner, P., M. Sutphen, V. Leonard, and L. Day. 2010. *Educating Nurses—A Call for Radical Transformation.* San Francisco, CA: Jossey-Bass.

Burns, P. 1991. "Elements of Spirituality and Watson's Theory of Transpersonal Caring: Expansion on Focus." In *Anthology on Caring.* P. L. Chinn, ed. New York: National League for Nursing Press.

Donner, G., and M. M. Wheeler. 2009. "Coaching in Nursing—An Introduction." http://donnerwheeler.com/documents/STTICcoaching.pd.

Hanson, C. 2011. "Interview with Nurse Practitioner Wellness Coaches." *Nurse Practitioner World News* 16(1): 7–9.

Health Ministries Association, Inc. April, 2010. "History of HMA—Twenty Years of Leadership." 1–3. http://www.hmassoc.org.

Hess, D., L. Bark, and M. E. Southard. 2010. "White Paper: Holistic Nurse Coaching." http://wellcoach.com/images/ WhitePaperHolisticNurseCoaching.pdf.

International Parish Nurse Resource Center (IPNRC). www. parishnurses.org/.

Luck, S. 2010. "Changing the Health of Our Nation—The Role of Nurse Coaches." *Alternative Therapies* 16(5): 78–80.

Luck, S., B. Dossey, and B. Schaub. 2011. "Holistic Nurse Coach Leadership Can Transform Healthcare." American Holistic Nurses Association. *Beginnings* 31(1): 8–10.

"Men in Nursing." Jan., 2005. Hodes Research. 38–135. www.hodes.com/resource/library.

Moore, M., and B. Tschannen-Moran. 2010. *Coaching Psychology Manual.* Philadelphia: Wolters Kluwer-Lippincott Williams & Wilkins.

Nelms, T. 1990. "The Lived Experience of Nursing Education: A Phenomenological Study." In Leininger, M., and J. Watson. *The Caring Imperative in Education.* New York: National League of Nursing.

Nepo, M. 2000. *The Book of Awakening.* San Francisco, CA: Conari Press.

Nepo, M. 2007. *Finding Inner Courage.* San Francisco, CA: Conari Press.

Newman, M. 2002. "The Pattern That Connects." *Advances in Nursing Science* 24(3): 1–7.

Newman, M. 2012. Health As Expanding Conciousness. http://www.healthasexpandingconsciousness.org/home/.

Roach, Simone. 1997 *Caring from the Heart—The Convergence of Caring and Spirituality.* Mahwah, NJ: Paulist Press.

Robert Wood Johnson Foundation. Sept. 28, 2011. "Human Capital: Male Nurses Break through Barriers to Diversify Profession." 1–2. http://www.rwfj.org/humancapital/product.jsp?id=72856.

Robert Wood Johnson Foundation. Aug., 2011. *Charting Nursing's Future: Implementing the IOM Future of Nursing Report Part 1:* "How to Dramatically Increase the Formal Education of America's Nursing Workforce by 2020." 1–7. www.nap.edu/catalog/12956.html.

Schenk, S., and K. Hartley. July–Sept., 2002. "Nurse Coach: Healthcare Resource for This Millenium." *Nursing Forum* 37(3): 14–20.

Wellness Initiative for the Nation (WIN). 2009. Samueli Institute. http://www.siib.org/news/new-home/WIN-Home.html.

Westberg, G. E. 2010. *Good Grief.* Fiftieth anniversary gift edition. Augsberg Fortress.

http://store.augsburgfortress.org/store/contributor/120/Granger+E.+Westberg

Westberg, G. E. 1991. *The Parish Nurse: Providing a Minister of Health for Your Congregation.* Augsberg Fortress. http://store.augsburgfortress.org/store/contributor/120/Granger+E.+Westberg.

This quote comes from Kay Donnelly, R.N., a nursing instructor in the 1970s: "Nursing gives you the opportunity to impact thousands (if not millions) of lives by simply caring. It is like being a rainbow in someone else's cloud." — Gail, R.N., 40 years

This quote comes from <u>Tao Te Ching</u>, New English version:
"The Master has no possessions,
The more she does for others,
The happier she is.
The more she gives to others,
The wealthier she is."
— Jeanine, R.N., M.S.N., 36 years

More than anything, I can say that there are times I could do nothing else but play the harp. We really bonded, my harp and I, because it was about the only thing in the whole world I felt somewhat sane and comforted by, and to be able not only to hear such beautiful melodies and harmony but to actually create them when I wanted to was an unspeakable blessing. One of the last memories I have of my dad is sitting at the piano bench together while he gave me some lessons on the piano and my harp. This is absolutely priceless to me, and I feel closest to him now when I play. — Marian, R.N., M.S.N., AHN-BC, 29 years

If nothing ever changed, there would be no butterflies—and of course butterflies are for courage and strength.They are daily life lessons for me and even now quoted by my grandchildren. — Pat, R.N., 19 years

7

PALLIATIVE MUSIC WITH HARP—
A JOURNEY TO EMBRACE
THE HEART OF NURSING

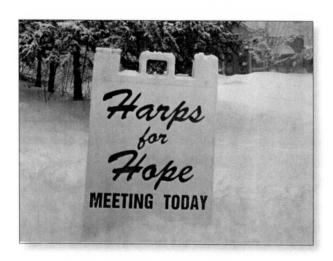

*My path in life is to be a spark, a light bearer,
and a seed planter.*

YVONNE FETIG ROEHLER

THE SPARK

We never know when the lens through which we see our role as nurses will widen to reveal a new spark of possibility. Twenty-plus years ago, I could not have fathomed that playing my harp at the bedside for Estyln, whose smiling face graces the dedication page, would lead me to write this closing chapter.

I began playing the folk harp in 1987 as an attempt at my own self-care while working as a hospice nurse. Initially, playing the harp became my way to temporarily distance myself from the emotional overload of intensive statewide work I was involved in to help both current and emerging hospice programs meet Michigan's hospice licensure requirements. At the same time I was completing my doctoral program research. Holding my small harp and gently plucking the strings resonated deep within to replenish the well of my soul. The harp also helped me renew intimacy with my "best self" while clarifying what was essential for my own healing and wellness.

That "stepping back" for emotional distance and perspective helped me to more confidently stride forward five years later to begin playing for patients and families in local hospice programs, nursing homes, and hospitals. It could be said that when I initially left the bedside, it was to learn how to come back to it more fully as a nurse with harp in hand.

A research study, perhaps one of the first of its kind, "The Effects of Live Music [singing and guitar playing] Versus Tape Recorded Music on Hospitalized Cancer Patients," was published in 1983 encouraging support for the "human element and caring presence." We have traveled quite a distance from these early findings, which report that "It is becoming increasingly evident that music can provide both physical and emotional comfort to hospitalized cancer patients. It is not fully understood why music is so beneficial to patients, although it is probably in part due to the effects that music has on the physiological process and the reduction of anxiety" (Bailey 17).

A Light

A glimmer of light began to shine with possibility when I discovered the impressive work of Therese Schroeder-Sheker, who began the field of Music Thanatology, a program of study that attends to the terminally ill and dying for the express purpose of "prescriptive musical care." Her Chalice of Repose project as recounted in "Music for the Dying" offered a two-year educational program that prepared participants to play harps and sing ancient Cluniac music at the bedside in teams of two for the terminally ill and actively dying patients.

The more I learned about the benefits of this wonderful expression of caring, the more firmly I believed it should not be limited to dying patients. It could even be used during pregnancy, childbirth, and neonatal care (Olson, "Bedside Musical Care," 572). However, I was still searching for a way to make my vision a reality.

The "way" was clearly illuminated in 1995 when I attended a weekend "modal music" workshop taught by Liz Cifani with my friend and nurse colleague Anne Hughes. In addition to her responsibilities as harpist with the Chicago Symphony Orchestra, Liz was also teaching a therapeutic and improvisational technique using musical modes with her harp. This method was easy to learn and did not require extensive knowledge or experience with music performance. It was the key I had been searching for that would open the door as a healing technique for bedside musical caring with harp.

Musical Modes

After silence, that which comes nearest to expressing the inexpressible is music.

Aldous Huxley, *Music at Night*

Ancient Greek modes were named for the tribes of peoples who migrated through the ancient empire from 1,230–1,050 B.C. The two major tribes were the Ionians from Asia Minor and the Aeolians from the island of Lesbos. Perhaps one of the most well known musicians who helped devise the particular sequences of modes was Pythagoras of Samos, the sixth-century philosopher, mathematician, and musician. He devised tonal sequences on the seven-string lyre with each string supposedly echoing one of the seven planets. The seven modes as we know them today are the Ionian, Dorian, Phrygian, Lydian, Lesbian (Mixolydian), Aeolian, and Locrian (Gardner 132).

In 1998, I subsequently proposed the following initial principles as the rationale for bringing music to the bedside:

♦ Music holistically affects the healing process even though a cure may not be possible

♦ Music potentially can bring profound humanness to the clinical environment for a wide range of patients across their life span and with varied health needs

♦ The qualities of vibratory tone, rhythm, pitch, and volume potentially affect the healing process

♦ Musical care by its very nature involves validation of the patient and the moment

♦ Musical care utilizes four realms of listening— the person, the environment, the self, and the spiritual space

We know that nearly every system of our body works on the principle of rhythm. Maintenance of these rhythms is essential in helping to ensure our optimal state of health and wellness. It is interesting that the word "per-son" literally means "the sound passes through." We are vibratory beings. Music can assist us with re-connecting and balancing the rhythms of our bodies and ultimately even the rhythm of our lives. Thus, whenever possible, two bedside harpers position themselves on each side of the bed to encourage optimal receptivity of the musical influence.

Musical modes also relate to the body's seven energy centers (chakras). What follows is a brief overview of each specific mode and its relationship to chakra location, spiritual aspects, basic needs, and positive emotions.

Mode	Chakra	Spiritual Aspect	Basic Needs	Positive Emotions
Ionian-C	base/root	self-awareness	belonging	courage
Dorian-D	below navel	self-respect	inter-dependence	nurturance
Phrigian-E	stomach	self-worth	self-esteem	confidence
Lydian-F	heart	self-love	unconditional love	joy
Mixolydian-G	throat	self-expression	change and let go	freedom
Aolian-A	between eyes	self-respon-sibility	purpose	wisdom, clarity
Lochrian-B	crown	self-knowing	acceptance	peace, humility

The significance of the number seven is quite evident. We have seven modes, seven chakras, and seven circuits of the labyrinth. Now, Robert Ferré in *The Labyrinth Revival* suggests that the patterns of the seven circuits are also linked musically by mathematical proportions as noted below (26):

On the scale of C, the paths are assigned these notes:

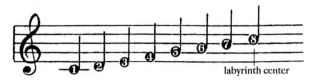

One possible melody for the seven-circuit labyrinth is this:

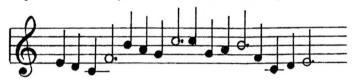

In his book *Sounds of Healing*, the physician and author Mitchell Gaynor stresses the importance of song transculturally to mark life cycle events. Through his reflections on the patients who came to him each day for cancer treatment and other ailments, he found a common thread: "It was not the specifics of their disease, but rather their inability to hear their personal life song. Their life experiences had caused them to become tone-deaf to the true and unencumbered voice of their own souls. Odd as it may seem, many of us unconsciously prefer to ignore the summons of our innermost essence" (34).

With regard to the term "compassion fatigue," could it be said that nurses experiencing consistently high levels of work stress become increasingly tone deaf to the harmony of their souls as they struggle to re-tune their priorities for self-care? It is an ominous vital sign indeed when nurses are unable to find the pulse of their own wellness.

In "Opening, Listening, and Caring through the Strings of a Harp," Amy Colombo details the beginning and subsequent growth of a therapeutic harp program at Munson Medical Center in Traverse City, Michigan, that now extends into hospice services and new program development with an affiliate hospital. Together, Amy and I co-teach both beginning and advanced palliative music with harp classes that are open to any hospital employee. Nurses also receive continuing education credits for their participation. More than anything, the participants have an opportunity to immerse themselves in a different perspective of what caring involves. Many take the class just to honor the importance of regaining balance with work and self.

Amy poignantly expresses the collective sentiment for our work this way: "The essence of modal music with the harp is that it permits me to come simply with what I have. This simplicity and sense of being unencumbered allows me to be open to what the patient needs, to listen in every sense of the word, and to fully care through the music, the vibrations, and the sound" (133).

PLANTING SEEDS OF WELLNESS
FOR THE COMMUNITY

In 2000, the seed for my ongoing community service was planted by a courageous young woman whom I met while playing for patients receiving outpatient chemotherapy. We saw each other frequently, and Catherine always shared how eager she was to get better and learn to play "that kind of music" with her own small harp. Sadly, her condition worsened, and while she was in the hospital, Catherine asked her good friend to take her harp to my office with the request that I "Make it sing for other women."

After work, I went immediately to the hospital and played Catherine's harp for her. Holding her hand, I whispered my deep gratitude and assured her that I would indeed make her harp, now named "Catherine," sing for other women. Although verbally unresponsive and with her eyes closed, she squeezed my hand. Catherine died later that evening. Embracing my promise to her, I taught my first community volunteer Heart to Harp class on the day of her funeral.

Since 2004, I have been offering a free community Harps for Hope class for men and women who are facing difficult life situations. Participants meet for six weeks to learn modal music on a small harp that is loaned to them for the duration of the class. Our focus is on playing modes for healing and self-care while also re-connecting again with a sense of wellness "from the inside out." It is always my hope that participants hear once again their own life songs through the modes of the harp, as expressed in the story shared by a recent participant in the class:

> It is difficult for me to put into words what it has meant to take this class and learn to play Catherine. Even at home, when I just look at the harp sitting by my chair, I feel this healing over my heart. I have a lot of healing to do in recovering from a poor relationship with my mother. Despite the fact that I have cared for her in my home for many years, she is unable to express any gratitude or love for me, a situation that began in my early childhood when nothing I did was ever good enough.
>
> When I started playing the harp, I felt like something opened up inside of me and for the first time I could forgive her. She won't change, but now I know that I do have something worthwhile to offer myself for healing—I am better than "good enough" for me. I believe in myself again.

As previously discussed in Chapter Four, nurses have the privilege of entering and honoring patients' spiritual space with their harps, most often at a very vulnerable time in patients' lives. Our presence with the harps validates their journey and the sacredness of the moment. However brief, we remain mindful of the breadth and depth of this experience. This focus is best described by James Miller and Susan Cutshall in their book *The Art of Being a Healing Presence*:

- *Intention*—beyond ourselves, to the greater good, to healing, to the sacredness of the moment, to and for the other, while letting go of personal expectations

- *Opening*—to the moment, to ourselves, to possibility, to healing, to courage, to acceptance of what is

- *Honoring*—clearing space and time, preparing, respecting, calming, quieting

- *Offering*—unselfish focus, simplicity, authenticity, presence, love, belief in possibilities, hope, unconditional regard, equality, humanness, separateness, sacredness

- *Receiving*—accepting the beauty and power of the moment as well as revelations, insight, lessons, peace

- *Balancing*—possibilities, solitude, action, inaction, affirmation, transformation, self, others

- *Stillness*—being open to reflection, peace, wisdom, gratitude, humility, transformation, validation, joy, growth (74–75)

It is indeed serendipitous that here we receive seven ways of being linked once again to the seven circles of the labyrinth.

CONCLUSION

I know this book may not appeal to every nurse. However, you are here with me now, and I am very grateful for your willingness to enter the deeperer water of caring with me. Thank you for your courage.

Nursing is truly more than a skill. It is living art, and both are needed within the circle of healing. I have witnessed nurses participating in the modal music harp classes who visibly soften their demeanor with self and others as they deepen and affirm their awareness of how to be a healing presence. The harp is simply their own voice musically helping them once again to reveal their spark within to be both a light bearer and a seed planter for compassion.

I conclude this chapter with a short song I wrote entitled "Every Nurse Matters." Share it with others if you like, knowing that the word "nurse" can also be substituted for people important to you.

Finally, I offer this blessing to each of you now and into your future remarkable life as a nurse:

May you arise each morning hearing the gentle harmony between your soul and your life.

SHARON OLSON, MAY 18, 2012

Every Nurse Matters

©Sharon Olson, 1994

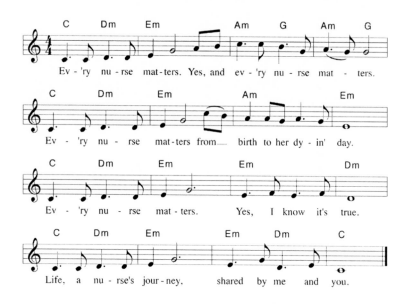

You may substitute "patient," "family," "volunteer," "woman," "man," "mother," "father," "sister," "brother," "grandmother," "grandfather," etc. in place of "nurse" for additional verses.

References

Bailey, L. 1983. "The Effects of Live Music Versus Tape-Recorded Music on Hospitalized Cancer Patients." *Music Therapy* 3(1): 17–28.

Colombo, A. 2012. "Opening, Listening, and Caring through the Strings of a Harp." In *Your Gift: An Educational, Spiritual, and Personal Resource for Hospice Volunteers.* Sharon Olson, ed. Traverse City, MI: Seasons Press.

Gardner, K. 1990. *Sounding the Inner Landscape—Music As Medicine.* Rockport, MA: Element Books.

Ferré, R. 1998. *The Labyrinth Revival.* St. Louis, Missouri: One Way Press.

Gaynor, M. 1999. *Sounds of Healing, A Physician Reveals the Therapeutic Power of Sound, Voice, and Music.* New York: Broadway Books.

Miller, J., and S. Cutshall. 2001. *The Art of Being a Healing Presence.* Fort Wayne, IN: Willowgreen Publications.

Olson, S. Sept./Oct. 1998. "Bedside Musical Care: Applications in Pregnancy, Childbirth, and Neonatal Care." *Journal of Gynecologic and Neonatal Nursing* 27(5): 569–575.

Schroeder-Sheker, T. Winter, 1994. "Music for the Dying: A Personal Account of the New Field of Music Thanatology—History, Theories, and Clinical Narratives." *Journal of Holistic Nursing* 12(1): 83–99.

Additional Resources
and Suggested Readings

Fox, M. 1979. *A Spirituality Named Compassion*. Minneapolis: Winston Press.

Harp Therapy Journal. www.harptherapy.com.

Kornfield, J. 2002. *The Art of Forgiveness, Loving Kindness, and Peace*. New York: Bantam.

Ladner, L. 2004. *The Lost Art of Compassion—Discovering the Practice of Happiness in the Meeting of Buddhism and Psychology*. New York: Harper One.

Roach, S. 1992. *The Human Act of Caring: A Blueprint for Health Professions*. Ottowa, Ontario: Canadian Hospital Association.

Sound and Music Alliance (SAMA). www.soundandmusic-alliance.org.

Watson Caring Science Institute International Caritas Consortium. www.watsoncaringscience.org.

ABOUT THE AUTHOR

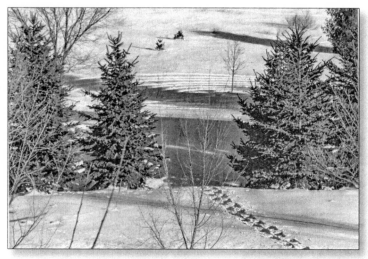

Labyrinth in winter

Sharon Olson, Ph.D., GNP-BC, relates that she has been on a lifelong learning curve that began in 1967 when she graduated from Trinity Hospital School of Nursing in Minot, North Dakota, with her cherished diploma in nursing. Since then, she has not stopped working and learning, seeking her B.S.N., a master's degree in both community service and nursing, and a Ph.D. in family ecology from Michigan State University.

After completing her Ph.D. in 1987, she worked as an associate professor at the University of Wisconsin-Stout campus in Menomonie, Wisconsin, where she taught a variety of courses focused on the family. In 1995, she and her husband John moved back to Michigan, settling on the beautiful Old Mission Peninsula, where Sharon completed her nurse practitioner degree. She subsequently began Partners in Prevention, focusing on rural health for elders and palliative care.

In 2006, her husband Dr. John Schneider, a clinical psychologist, joined the practice and together they developed a mutual treatment focus of wellness and healing. In that year, Sharon was highlighted in the MSU College of Nursing "60 Years of Distinction" calendar identifying alumni who embraced the heart of nursing. She was also acknowledged by Nursing Spectrum as a regional award winner for her community service.

Sharon now dedicates the remainder of her nursing career to the well-being both of nursing students and nurses in the firm belief that to offer caring for others first requires mindfully and consistently walking a path for your own self-care. She acknowledged the need for her own self-care in 1987 when she began playing the folk harp to temporarily distance herself from the emotional overload and intense involvement of her hospice work. In that distancing process, she found a new healing source that she subsequently brought to the bedside for others.

Over half of Sharon's nursing career has involved education, support, and promotion for expanding hospice care in Michigan. Her authorship of three edited editions of *Your Gift: An Educational, Spiritual, and Personal Resource for Hospice Volunteers* spans twenty-five years. In great measure, hospice care became the inspiration and exemplar for her ecological model of wellness for nurses.

NOTES

NOTES

NOTES

NOTES

Notes

CPSIA information can be obtained at www.ICGtesting.com
Printed in the USA
BVOW031341080812

297323BV00001B/2/P